CBT FOR
OLDER PEOPLE

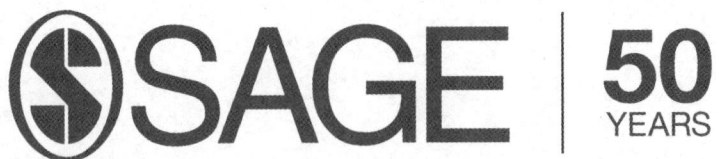

SAGE was founded in 1965 by Sara Miller McCune to support the dissemination of usable knowledge by publishing innovative and high-quality research and teaching content. Today, we publish more than 750 journals, including those of more than 300 learned societies, more than 800 new books per year, and a growing range of library products including archives, data, case studies, reports, conference highlights, and video. SAGE remains majority-owned by our founder, and after Sara's lifetime will become owned by a charitable trust that secures our continued independence.

Los Angeles | London | Washington DC | New Delhi | Singapore

CBT FOR OLDER PEOPLE

AN INTRODUCTION

KEN LAIDLAW

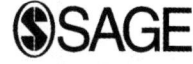

Los Angeles | London | New Delhi
Singapore | Washington DC

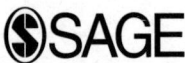

Los Angeles | London | New Delhi
Singapore | Washington DC

SAGE Publications Ltd
1 Oliver's Yard
55 City Road
London EC1Y 1SP

SAGE Publications Inc.
2455 Teller Road
Thousand Oaks, California 91320

SAGE Publications India Pvt Ltd
B 1/I 1 Mohan Cooperative Industrial Area
Mathura Road
New Delhi 110 044

SAGE Publications Asia-Pacific Pte Ltd
3 Church Street
#10-04 Samsung Hub
Singapore 049483

Editor: Kate Wharton
Assistant editor: Laura Walmsley
Production editor: Rachel Burrows
Copyeditor: Dan Harding
Proofreader: Bryan Campbell
Indexer: Bill Farrington
Marketing manager: Camille Richmond
Cover design: Wendy Scott
Typeset by: C&M Digitals (P) Ltd, Chennai, India
Printed in Great Britain by Henry Ling Limited at
The Dorset Press, Dorchester, DT1 1HD

Library of Congress Control Number: 2014941226

British Library Cataloguing in Publication data

A catalogue record for this book is available from
the British Library

MIX
Paper from
responsible sources
FSC
www.fsc.org   FSC™ C013985

ISBN 978-1-84920-459-0
ISBN 978-1-84920-460-6 (pbk)

At SAGE we take sustainability seriously. Most of our products are printed in the UK using FSC papers and boards.
When we print overseas we ensure sustainable papers are used as measured by the Egmont grading system.
We undertake an annual audit to monitor our sustainability.

Contents

About the Author

Professor Ken Laidlaw is Head of the Department of Clinical Psychology and Programme Director of the ClinPsyD Clinical Psychology Training Programme within the Norwich Medical School, at the University of East Anglia. Professor Laidlaw is also currently honorary consultant clinical psychologist with Norfolk and Suffolk NHS Trust, having for many years served as Professional Lead of an Older Adult Clinical Psychology Service in Scotland. He maintains active and ongoing research activity in cognitive behaviour therapy (CBT) for late life depression and anxiety, especially with complex, chronic and comorbid conditions. From 2000 to 2001 he was invited to spend a year at the University of Pennsylvania (PENN) in Philadelphia with Aaron T. Beck, the father of CBT, as visiting scholar. He has a long and productive association with Professors Larry W. Thompson and Dolores Gallagher-Thompson at Stanford University, California, USA. He was the Principal Investigator on the first UK RCT of CBT for late life depression. His manual for this trial has subsequently been used in other clinical trials. He also led the development of a cross-cultural Attitudes to Ageing Questionnaire (AAQ), that was piloted and field trialled in 20 countries worldwide. This is now used widely in international trials. His conceptualisation framework for CBT with older people is part of the UK's Increasing Access to Psychological Therapies (IAPT) initiative, and informs the IAPT curriculum materials for HI IAPT workers. He authored the older adults section of the evidence-based guide to the commissioning of psychological therapies for the NHS in Scotland (*The Psychology Matrix*, NES, 2011).

Acknowledgements

I want to acknowledge the great generosity of all my clients in allowing me to learn with them when facing their current life challenges and I am very grateful to those who agreed to have some of their stories shared for training purposes. The clients I worked with always showed great resilience and tenacity in facing problems with a strength of character forged from adversity that always impresses and inspires me, even if they sometimes found it very hard to give themselves much credit for what they did. I hope to have gained some important insights as a result that I can pass on in this text.

I am also indebted to the editorial team at Sage, Kate and Laura in particular showed me the greatest patience in waiting for this book to be finished. They never seemed to give up on this book, and were always positive and supportive. I am so very grateful they kept their faith in me. I could not have hoped for a better team to work with.

Finally, I am fortunate to have an amazing support system at home. My wife Mary and our daughter Katherine were very forgiving of the time I took away from family tasks in order to write. I dedicate this book to them in love and gratitude.

PART 1

Preparing to Use CBT with Older People

One

Introduction to CBT

Learning Objectives
By the end of this chapter you will:

- Have increased your understanding of the Beck model of psychopathology
- Understand why therapists need to use CBT theory in order to be more skilled and flexible in applying CBT
- Be introduced to the idea that while CBT has an elegantly simple model, the application of CBT requires discipline and practice
- Understand the basic structure of a course of CBT-based treatment for depression or anxiety

What is CBT?

Cognitive behaviour therapy (CBT) with older people is a mainstream treatment approach for the alleviation of depression and anxiety in later life. It is particularly appropriate as an intervention for older adults because it is skills enhancing, present-oriented, problem focused, straightforward to use and effective (Laidlaw et al., 2003).

Central to CBT for people with depression or anxiety is the concept that an individual's appraisal of their experience, rather than the experience itself, is what determines its impact. A useful way of helping your client to understand that there are different ways to think about any situation is to introduce your client to optical illusions. Optical illusions illustrate the idea that every experience is perceived uniquely and idiosyncratically. Thus, when we have a thought about an event or an experience our thoughts are just one of many different interpretations from an abundance of possibilities, and what gives an experience its impact on us individually is not the character of that event, but the meanings and significance ascribed to it. This idea is quite subtle, as many people assume that our thoughts can be the only way to look at something. Visual illusions show us this is not the case.

Figure 1.1 is a classic visual illusion drawn by the cartoonist W.E. Hill based on postcards dating from the nineteenth century. Published in 1915 in the magazine *Puck*, it is known as 'My wife and mother-in-law'. It is an ambiguous illusion, and as

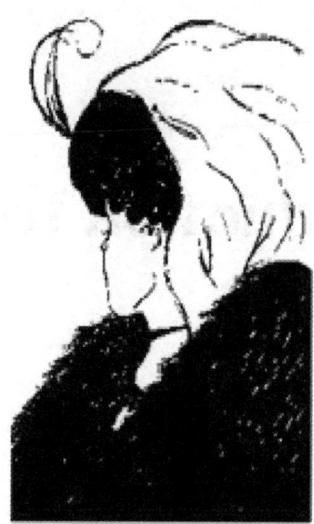

FIGURE 1.1   *Visualising CBT*

such the 'data' may be resolved in different, but equally valid, ways. Thus, when you ask your client to look at this figure and ask what they see, you can discuss not only whether they see an old woman or a young woman, but you can discuss the way our minds make sense of ambiguous data. In the cognitive behavioural approach to understanding the impact of thoughts on feelings and behaviour this is an important explanatory concept. It is the way we see things that is important, and just because we see things in a certain way this does not mean it is the only way to view things. If we think something that does not make it a fact or any more correct than the way someone else will see a situation. It really is *in the eye of the beholder.* Figure 1.1 provides us with an example of how we might make sense of things in one way, but there are often many more ways to view a situation – hence the reason we consider our thoughts in CBT.

The Beck CBT model as it applies to depression is beguilingly simple, but one of the first challenges to becoming a skilled cognitive therapist is to understand that simple ideas require discipline and practice. The connection between thought, mood and behaviour seems so simple and self-evident that it can come as quite an unpleasant surprise when your clients do not instantly get better or their cognitions become difficult to challenge and modify. This book aims to equip you with a realistic appraisal of CBT.

The techniques and ideas contained in this book are the product of the author's many years' experience studying and practicing. If you as the therapist approach CBT as a simple concept this will wrong-foot you from the start, as CBT requires discipline, skill, perseverance and great patience.

While there are many 'cookbook' guides to applying CBT, these can sometimes be unhelpful as they suggest a simplicity of approach incompatible with an idiosyncratically delivered treatment programme that is much more than a collection of techniques and tools. CBT explicitly sets out to understand the person's world, and a full understanding can only be achieved through careful and deliberate exploration augmented with a methodology that emphasises a 'test it out' approach. CBT educates, motivates and challenges the person to bring about symptom change.

Techniques do not make a therapy work however, *people do*, and it is in the sympathetic and skilled application of techniques allied to a good therapeutic treatment alliance that CBT becomes an effective and powerful treatment intervention for late life depression and anxiety. CBT aims to be empowering of individuals and seeks to promote self-agency, as it adopts a non-pathologising stance to understanding how a client's problems may have developed (Zeiss & Steffen, 1996). As such, it can be a very attractive form of therapy for older people who often endorse strong cohort beliefs about personal independence and problem solving. To do CBT well requires great skill and ingenuity – one must be scientific, approachable and accessible. The goal is for clients to become their own therapists.

CBT can be differentiated from other forms of psychotherapy as:

- Sessions are structured according to an explicit agenda
- Collaborative empiricism is emphasised throughout treatment
- Negative interpretations are hypotheses requiring empirical testing (thoughts aren't facts and are open to disputation)
- Homework tasks are essential to generalise learning outside of the session and to promote an enhanced sense of agency
- The primary means of exploration is Socratic questioning, although ...
- CBT is a 'doing cure' as much as, if not more than, a 'talking cure' (enduring change comes from the client doing things differently). Nevertheless ...
- CBT assumes that behaviour change will also bring about cognitive change
- Interventions are linked to individualised case-conceptualisations

It is of course recommended that you seek out supervision from an experienced cognitive behaviour therapist when applying CBT as your main treatment approach in your workplace. You may wish to look at the website of the British Association of Behavioural and Cognitive Psychotherapists (BABCP: www.babcp.com) to learn more about the requirements for competence in the practice of CBT.

Starting now, think about what you know about CBT and what you want to know. This is a useful technique to figure out the gaps in your knowledge. It can also be useful to write down your beliefs and then test them out later by trying to find evidence for and against them. Doing this exercise gives you a small insight into the types of tasks we ask our clients to do. Use the worksheet here.

What do I know about CBT?	
Things I like and understand	Things I don't like or don't understand
Gaps in my knowledge	Ways to address these (✓) ☐ Further study/CPD ☐ Specific reading ☐ Supervision ☐ Complete CTRS ☐ Share CTRS with someone ☐ Go to workshops ☐ Find a mentor
Gaps in my competence	Ways to address these (✓) ☐ Further study/CPD ☐ Specific reading ☐ Supervision ☐ Complete CTRS ☐ Share CTRS with someone ☐ Go to workshops ☐ Find a mentor

Once you complete the worksheet, set yourself a homework task to achieve over the next week based on how you have completed the form. It should be linked to the task in hand, so perhaps you might like to read a specific article about the theory of CBT, or alternatively you might like to read a paper on a specific technique or aspect of therapy. Once you have completed your homework task, write a few notes about what you have learned.

Note: if you engage in this task, not only will you learn a bit more about CBT, you will be learning something about the process behind it. You will learn what it feels like to embark on a homework assignment and hopefully how good it feels when you learn something new or unexpected.

The Aaron T. Beck Model of CBT

In this book the form of CBT utilised draws mainly upon that developed by Aaron T. Beck (see Beck et al., 1979; Beck, 1983; Beck 2008). In this book, the philosophical orientation of the author is to appreciate that talking can be helpful and important in helping clients understand and address problems, but in order to bring about enduring change, therapy needs to be more than a 'talking cure' – it needs to be a 'doing cure'.

Thus, behaviour experiments are vital if you want your clients to bring about real and lasting change in their lives and, as Garratt et al. (2007) note, the cognitive model assumes that behaviour change facilitates changes in cognitive structures (schemata). In this way behavioural and cognitive interventions are likely to be necessary to bring about improvement in dysphoria.

The mechanism of change in Beck's model remains somewhat elusive. While Beck (1976) originally proposed that CBT brought about a fundamental change in dysfunctional schemata following treatment, this has been under scrutiny and alternative suggestions are that dysfunctional schemata become deactivated following successful treatment, or that compensatory schemata are developed that reduce the impact of existing schemata and mental models (Garratt et al., 2007). Whatever theory you prefer, it is clear that successful treatment in CBT can be a profound experience for your client as they develop new ways of interacting with, and understanding, the world.

The schematic in Figure 1.2 provides a representation of Beck's cognitive model of psychopathology. The model provides therapists with a way of describing the nature of the presentation of their client but also a way to predict future challenges in the therapeutic process.

Notice that it actually operates on two levels: the overt level (which is often the symptom level and the more overt thoughts, feelings and behaviour associated with distress) and the covert level (schemata etc.). The covert level is the underlying belief structure or core values of an individual. Note that an individual may be unaware that their beliefs are maladaptive and ultimately self-defeating.

The Beck model is a stress–diathesis model (Garratt et al., 2007; Liu & Alloy, 2010) that operates on two different levels. The first level is overt and it takes very little 'digging' on the part of the therapist to uncover the client's overt distress.

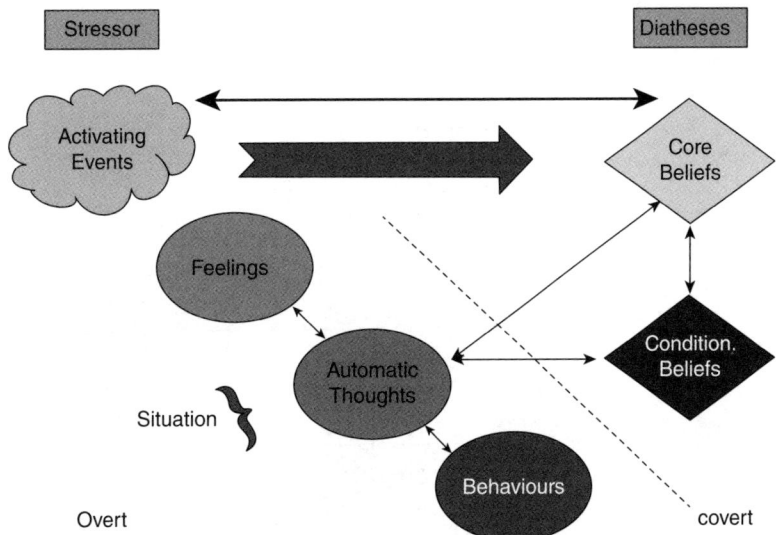

FIGURE 1.2 *Beck's model of psychopathology*

This is most commonly seen in the client's thoughts and is illustrated in Figure 1.2. Underlying the negative thoughts, at a covert level, are core beliefs, which may contribute to the themes evident in negative cognitions. This concept is illustrated in Figure 1.3.

The underlying covert level acts as the diathesis, usually activated by a linked stressor. This model may assume that the person is relatively passive and at the mercy of external events. This can be an oversimplification, as research suggests there may be a stress-generation process, as people with depression are likely to interact with stressors in a bidirectional manner (Liu & Alloy, 2010), in that people with depression may interact with stressors in a way that make it more likely that aversive experiences occur more frequently. This is a particularly troubling aspect of depression and anxiety symptoms – problems are magnified and multiplied by maladaptive responses.

Thus, it is usually important for therapists to ask themselves why the client is experiencing difficulties, what are the meanings they are ascribing to events and how may this be understood by considering the underlying maladaptive structure of *core beliefs*, *conditional beliefs* and *compensatory strategies*. Is there a reciprocal interaction between the individual, the stressors and their (over)reactions and (over)compensatory strategies? The structure of the Beck model is illustrated in Figure 1.4.

In the Beck model, thoughts are crucial for understanding the emotional reactions and behavioural responses in someone experiencing a depression. The schematic in Figure 1.4 can function as a useful conceptualisation diagram and is a useful format to use when sharing your thoughts with your client, especially if there is a theme or

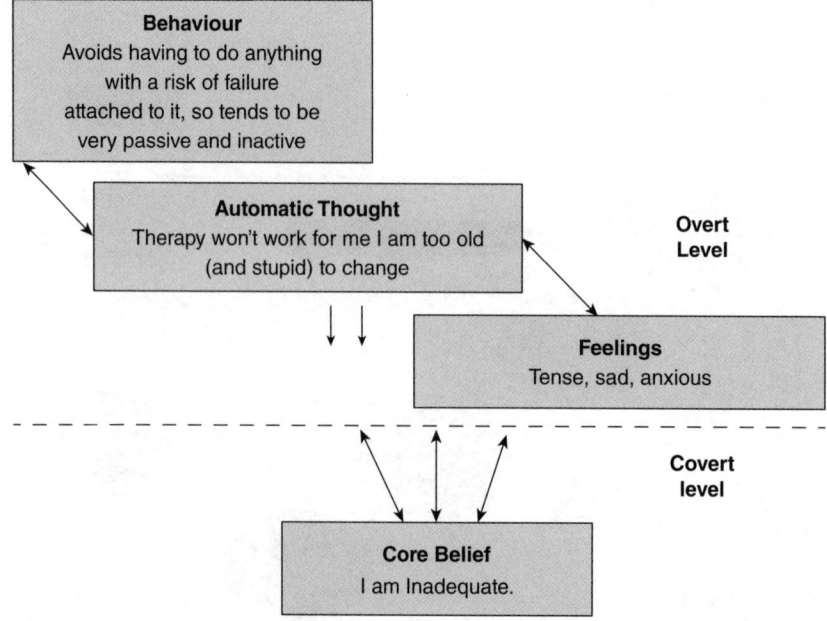

FIGURE 1.3 *Negative thoughts and their underlying covert structure*

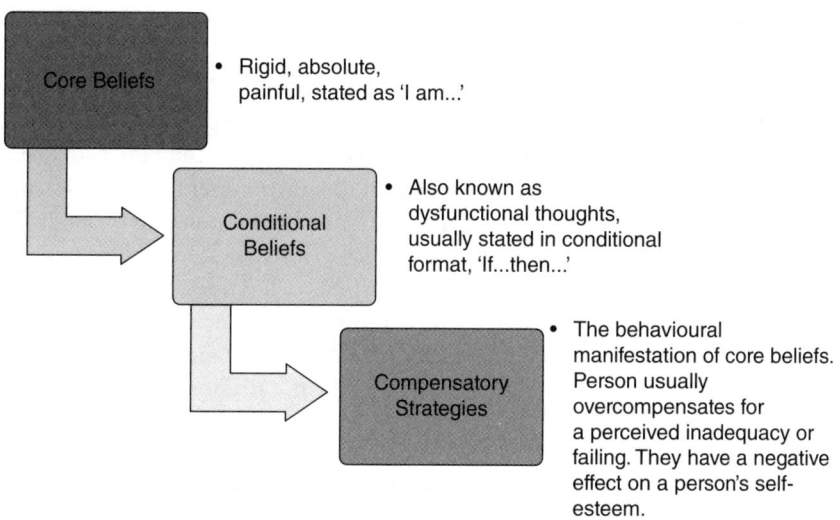

FIGURE 1.4   *The covert level of the Beck model of psychopathology*

unhelpful pattern of behaviours evident in your client's description of distressing events; there may be a pattern of overcompensating behaviours that can become self-defeating. In the chapter on conceptualisation, later in this book, there is a summary sheet for conceptualising all you understand about your client in terms of the Beck model. This sheet may also prove useful when feeding this back to your client (see Figure 8.5, p. 128).

An example of the application of the above model in Figures 1.3–1.5 may be illuminative here. When your client reports feeling depressed it is important to explore the *specific* thoughts they may be experiencing alongside this feeling, and the impact this has on their behaviour. For instance, thoughts may reflect some symptoms associated with depression such as hopelessness. So your client may think, 'this therapy isn't working for me, I'm too old to change'. Associated feelings may be sadness, anger and frustration (you may wish to ascertain the percentage strength of feeling associated with each of these emotions). In response, changes in behaviour will result in a further reduction of activity levels and your client may find it more difficult to persevere with their homework task (e.g. calling up a friend to meet for a coffee) as they feel hopeless about the possibility for change. They may even be experiencing a sense of hopelessness as they negatively ascribe problems to do with their age and think, 'What else did I expect ageing to be like, it's all downhill from here'. Each thought sets off a different emotional response and each thought can be linked to themes that are associated with the covert level of schema beliefs (Figure 1.4).

From this example, it may be seen that behaviour in depression can reinforce beliefs evident in negative automatic thoughts, and this can create a negative downward spiral that appears to confirm their thoughts as facts. Behaviours in depression are seen therefore as consequences of the negative automatic thoughts experienced in depression. Thought identification and psychoeducation about the cognitive theory of depression (e.g. mood congruent biases, negativity hypotheses, etc.) can be used to educate the person about the interaction of thoughts and feelings, but also to engage them in a dialogue about behaviour change in order to promote symptom change.

At the covert level, core beliefs may have been activated by a recent stressor congruent with pre-existing vulnerabilities (core beliefs), as in the stress–diathesis model. Core beliefs act like diatheses, and in the CBT model of psychopathology of Beck et al. (1979) the stress–diathesis is an important explanatory concept. The diatheses are idiosyncratic vulnerabilities that predispose an individual to develop depression if there are certain stresses evident in the environment. 'Cognitive vulnerability in the form of dysfunctional schemas and maladaptive personality are diatheses that remain latent in the non-depressed state until primed or activated by an eliciting event or stimulus' (Clark, Beck & Alford, 1999: 292). In a stress–diathesis there is a person–experience interaction, and depression may be explained by the activation of pre-existing vulnerabilities that confront an individual. These diatheses, or vulnerabilities, are often deemed to be latent until activated by the stressors in the environment experienced by the individual. In Figure 1.3 the connection between core beliefs and overt symptoms was identified. The covert structure of rigidly held, painful core beliefs maintains a painful and corrosive self-view that can become self-defeating and demoralising for your client. This is illustrated in Figure 1.5.

Core beliefs represent beliefs people hold to be true of themselves and are usually what we fear to be true of ourselves at our lowest most vulnerable times in our lives. Core beliefs are usually learned throughout development (and may be forged throughout the lifespan developmental process), and unlike negative thoughts they are much less amenable to change using diaries or thought restructuring.

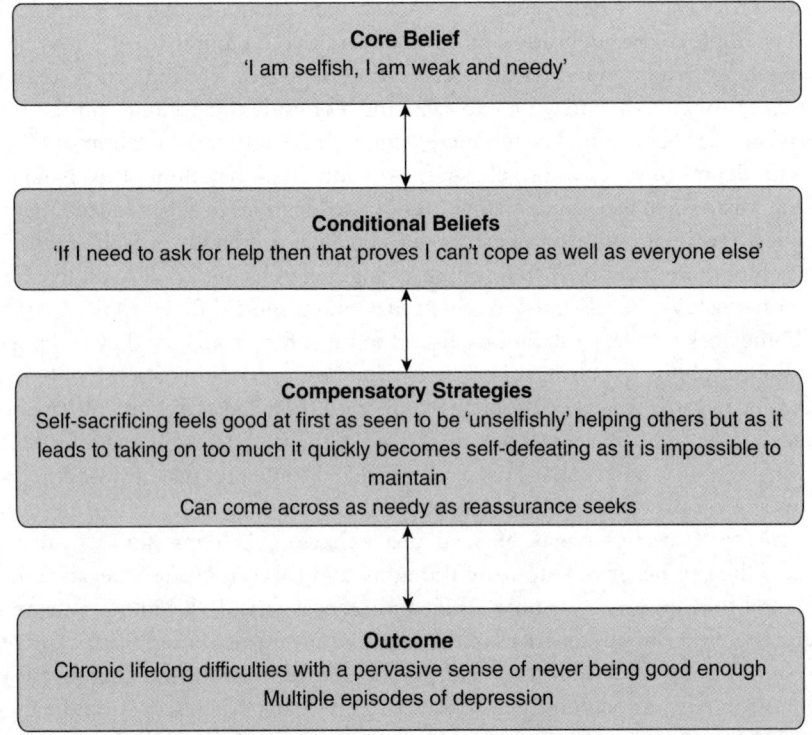

FIGURE 1.5   *Underlying maladaptive covert structure of beliefs in CBT*

Conditional beliefs are the core beliefs in action. They are called conditional beliefs as they are stated conditionally, i.e. in *'if…then'* terms (Figure 1.5). Conditional beliefs are also sometimes known as dysfunctional assumptions. As the maladaptive core belief and conditional belief structure can be very dysfunctional, the individual usually strives to maintain a level of functioning (holding down a job, raising a family, etc.) and therefore tends to engage in compensatory strategies (Beck, 2011). It is hard to get a balance with compensation, and as a result the person may be inclined to overcompensate especially in times of stress. This has the effect of undermining the individual's self-esteem as they find it difficult to get their needs recognised and met. Additionally, they often experience their compensatory strategies failing to work out for them or others in their life. Unless these are addressed the individual is often doomed to be the architect of their own problems.

Understanding how an individual makes sense of their experience means understanding them in context. This may be in the context of their relationships with others or their relationship with themselves. With older people this can often mean that CBT needs to be augmented by factors that influence people's experience of ageing. Psychotherapists working with older people require an understanding of gerontology to achieve this understanding (see also Laidlaw & McAlpine, 2008).

CBT provides the person with strategies and problem-solving skills to identify and challenge negative or unhelpful thought–feeling–behaviour interactions and habitual idiosyncratic maladaptive patterns of responding to situations. CBT utilises a systematic and creative process that needs to be delivered at the person's own pace.

At the start of treatment you need to be able to state what the *focus of treatment* is: are you using interventions to reduce anxiety, or are you using interventions to improve mood? Clearly interventions for anxiety are different than when the focus is depression, but they do sometimes overlap. Thus, if you are not careful you may end up becoming confused and lost in your treatment approach. Consult your conceptualisation/formulation: are you mainly adopting one for anxiety or depression, and is it adequate as a framework to guide your interventions? In CBT the content of thoughts are distinct (known as cognitive content specificity, see Beck & Perkins, 2001 for review) in that we ought to be able to discriminate depressive cognitive content from anxious cognitive content.

TABLE 1.1 *Cognitive specificity in depression and anxiety cognitions*

	Cognitive specificity	**Behavioural consequences**
Depression	In your CBT interventions aimed at reducing depression symptoms you ought to be able to identify themes in the cognitive content of your client revolving around shame and regret, loss, failure and hopelessness.	Isolation, disengagement and lowered activity levels.
Anxiety	In your CBT interventions aimed at reducing anxiety symptoms you ought to be able to identify themes in the cognitive content of your client revolving around danger, threat (catastrophes are common fears) and inadequacy to cope with demands.	Avoidance, agitation (due to enhanced focus on catastrophe), self-fulfilling actions if acting when highly anxious.

Beck and Perkins (2001) carried out an interesting review into the status of the cognitive content specificity hypotheses and found the evidence was strongest for depressive cognitive content specificity and less so for anxiety cognitive content. The authors provide an interesting alternative perspective, and that is to use *self-discrepancy theory* to differentiate depressed people from anxious people. In depression the discrepancy is between actual self and idealised self, whereas in anxiety the discrepancy is between actual self and ought self (see Beck & Perkins, 2001; Higgins, 1987). In this case, the 'ought self' comprises the personal attributes we ought to possess with regard to duty, obligations and responsibilities (Higgins, 1987). Interestingly, when working with older people an 'ought self' discrepancy that appears common is exemplified by the statement: 'at my age I ought to be able to cope on my own by now'. In this case the weight of the 'ought self' attribution can pile a lot of additional pressure onto people, and this can lead to shame and embarrassment on the part of your client. Be aware of this, as it may be so onerous that your client fails to return to your sessions.

> Whatever you do in CBT you need to be clear what symptoms you are focusing on and how congruent your interventions are in this case. Consider the actual-ideal and actual-ought self-discrepancy when listening to your client cognitions.

Assessing the Suitability of Older People for CBT

Clinicians mindful of the need to apply evidence-based treatments when resources are scarce, or when service developments promote matched or stepped care approaches to treatment, may ask what types of older people make suitable candidates for CBT. Currently it is impossible to answer this question on an individual basis as the person, their presenting problem, the context for their problems and other historical factors make it bewilderingly complex especially as there is very little accumulated evidence (Kingdon et al., 2007). It is accepted that CBT does not work for everyone, therefore suitability is an important topic to consider. Perhaps at an individual level you may be more capable of using it with some clients rather than with others, and therefore you may wish to consider what your own continuing education needs are.

The development of suitability criteria for CBT is most fully considered by Safran and Segal (1996), who developed a set of guidelines that predict which patients will be suitable for CBT. The Suitability for Short-Term Cognitive Therapy Rating Scale (SSCTS, Safran & Segal, 1996) is a therapist-rated short questionnaire providing a measure of suitability for CBT. The scale measures a patient's suitability in terms of their ability to access thoughts, awareness and differentiation of emotions, acceptance of personal responsibility for change, compatibility with cognitive rationale, alliance potential, chronicity of problems, use of security and safety-seeking operations and the ability to maintain a problem focus in therapy.

Although the SSCTS is very interesting and has been thoughtfully developed, taking account of process factors that influence outcome, if applied with older people it may potentially act as a barrier to CBT being offered for a number of reasons. For instance, when considering chronicity of problems, older people may have a long history of depression but no history of receiving psychotherapy. Likewise, if older people are unused to psychotherapy they may not wholeheartedly endorse the cognitive rationale, and generally the level of psychological mindedness of older people can be quite low, although as the baby boomer generation increasingly turns 65 this may become less of an issue.

In addition, security and safety-seeking operations in therapy are considered to occur when patients use 'tangential or circumlocutory talking that makes it difficult to deal with any one subject in depth' (Safran & Segal, 1996: 255). However, older people often engage in storytelling and may be inclined to talk tangentially when discussing problems or issues in therapy. This should not be considered to be security operations (i.e. a way of avoiding talking about shame-inducing or embarrassing issues or anxiety-inducing topics within therapy) on the part of older people in therapy, but is merely the 'elder statesman' storytelling mode that older generations adopt when talking with younger members of their family. When assisted, with empathy and warmth on the part of an active therapist, older people can talk very movingly and with intense and sustained focus about issues of shame, hurt and distress.

Used rigidly, all older people would be considered very poor candidates for CBT when applying the SSCTS. It is clear however, that this scale was not developed for use with older people, and the authors did not develop this scale to be used inflexibly, nor for this client group. Moreover, the authors stress the need for therapists to resist interpretation and instead focus on a phenomenological exploration of the patient's world. One cannot replace clinical judgement entirely with scales, and therefore the therapist should always examine the full picture when considering possible reasons for exclusion of access to psychological intervention.

The question of suitability should be considered from the point of view of the client in terms of how CBT can be made suitable for the particular needs of the client. In other words: how can older people *benefit* from therapy rather than whether they are an optimal fit for treatment using the CBT model?

Fry (1986) notes, in determining suitability of older people for CBT:

> Thus the question of whether the elderly are a good or a bad prospect for therapy cannot use age per se as a definitive criteria. The assessment depends first on the therapist's own values and frame of reference and second on the elderly client's special problems and concerns. (Fry, 1986: 258)

While this quote was published some time ago, it remains relevant and important.

Blenkiron (1999) argues that given the active problem–focused nature of CBT, clients who are more focused on a predefined set of problems are likely to make more specific and measureable gains. This has some common sense behind it, but clients who are less able to organise their thoughts may nonetheless make good candidates for CBT if the therapist takes a more systematic and consistent approach to the structure of sessions and a logical strategy to organising seemingly disparate aspects of a client's problem list.

The perspective ought to be finding inclusion criteria, as many older people struggle to be referred to a psychological therapist in the first place (Gum et al., 2006; Kuruvilla et al., 2006). For this reason alone, when considering suitability it is advocated that therapists adopt a collaboratively empirical stance with their patient over possible outcomes at the start. Until we have well-established robust criteria we ought to adopt collaborative empiricism with our clients and review progress frequently and openly. Collaborative empiricism in these circumstances means adopting a 'try it and see' approach. One can never know unless one tries.

Indeed, to explicitly state that one does not know whether CBT will work or will be suitable for the client's needs is to acknowledge that a *joint* process of discovery has begun. CBT is at its best when discoveries are made that facilitate new understandings on the part of the client and which the therapist also finds illuminating. Sometimes therapists can be astounded at the potential change clients can achieve and the resilience they may demonstrate in managing problems in later life (Blazer, 2010). Thus, suitability criteria can be considered but only as one element in a complex decision-making process that must include the client seeking help and the settings in which treatment takes place (Blenkiron, 1999). Suitability must also be bidirectional, in that the client must be able to say if they feel the therapist or the therapy being offered is not suitable for their needs.

Adaptation, Modification or Augmentation for CBT with Older People?

When applying CBT with older people, the usual issue that comes up is whether CBT needs to be adapted in order to achieve optimal outcome. This seems a fairly reasonable thing to consider, especially when working with clients whose problems have lasted longer than the therapist's own lifespan. There are fears about frailty, response to treatment and about how much a therapist can expect a client to progress in the face of age-related challenges. However, introducing new elements into CBT such as unstructured life-review, or adopting a more passive and accepting stance to problems of longevity, may be adaptations that dilute the efficacy of CBT. The problem with adapting CBT is that there is no current evidence that adaptations are necessary or improve outcome – nevertheless, therapists are entitled to ask: how is CBT different with older people?

The main differences in CBT with older versus younger people is in regard to increased levels of physical comorbidity with psychological problems (e.g. as a result of conditions such as stroke and post-stroke depression), chronicity as evidenced by a lifetime's experience of living with recurrent mental health problems (thus depression and anxiety in later life are usually not late onset but more probably recurrent) and age-specific lifespan developmental factors (e.g. cohort). Finally, social networks and hence social capital may reduce as one ages – loss is a fact of ageing, especially as people are living longer.

Regardless, many older people come into therapy for the same reasons that most adults of working age do: because of difficulty in negotiating and overcoming unwanted or unexpected transitions. Life is always full of change and challenge, and for many people change can be stressful, especially when an element of choice is not part of the equation. For many older people challenging transitions can revolve around loss of physical or psychological independence. Thus CBT may be different in regard to the types of challenges facing people as they age. The client will benefit from working with a therapist who has some experience in apprehending these types of challenges and problems, which means that CBT therapists need to understand normal and abnormal ageing as well as demographic changes in society. As older people may misattribute their problems as being global (all of their problems are because they are old), stable (these problems are to do with ageing and as such are with them for the rest of their life) and internal (an attribute of the individual, i.e. their age), therapists need to be able to counter this with knowledge, skills and competences that equip them to pursue an active and empowering agenda for increased personal agency in the face of ageing.

In the main, adaptations suggested for CBT with older people tend to be vague, poorly thought-out procedural recommendations in the absence of any evidence for their necessity that could encourage therapeutic drift from an evidence-based efficacious therapy (Laidlaw & McAlpine, 2008). To this author, adaptations suggest that something is not suited to the task or to the needs of a population. Therefore, to suggest that CBT needs to be adapted may implicitly suggest a therapist is seeing either CBT or the client group (in this case older people) as somehow deficient in some respects. Either CBT needs to be adapted in order that older people can benefit, or it suggests the therapist considers older people to be unable to access CBT in the standard form used in adult mental health settings. As older people represent a very heterogeneous population, chronological factors are the least compelling reasons for making adaptations to an efficacious therapy.

Suggested adaptations to CBT with older people have tended to focus on procedural elements that take account of age-related changes. Usual recommendations suggest slowing sessions down, encouraging repetition of information and ensuring that interviews take place in a quiet, well-ventilated, well-lit room (Grant & Casey, 1995; Zeiss & Steffen, 1996). While it is not argued here that these adaptations are wrong, or even unnecessary, they are relatively banal, as one might expect therapists to incorporate these elements in response to individual need.

As CBT is an individually tailored treatment intervention the issue of adaptation at an individual level becomes less of an issue, so long as the main structural and conceptual elements are retained in each session. Charlesworth and Greenfield (2004) recommend that any adaptations ought to be predicated on the basis of need not age. However, the issue isn't really one of adaptation but one of augmentation. Stated more simply, can CBT be made to work more efficaciously with older people? To potentially augment the efficacy of CBT may require conceptual adaptation, and gerontology may hold the key to successful augmentation. Relevant theories that may augment the efficacy of CBT with older people include: selection, optimisation with compensation, stereotype embodiment theory and wisdom. Other important augmentations may be to use more contemporary approaches to CBT with older people, such as the enhanced role of compassion as an important intervention within CBT. For more on this topic see Chapter 9.

Specialist Knowledge for Applying CBT with Older People?

Recently the Department of Health (NHS England) commissioned an indicative curriculum for IAPT practitioners who may come into contact with older people. This new curriculum, overseen by national UK experts in CBT and in consultation with older people, includes guidelines for training materials for therapists wishing to work with older people. These materials are available online at: www.iapt.nhs.uk/workforce/iapt-older-peoples-training and www.iapt.nhs.uk/equalities/older-people.

More internationally, there have been developments in outlining the competences and knowledge base required when working psychologically with older people. This has resulted in the development of a set of guidelines that can be accessed by consulting the website for the council of professional geropsychology training programmes, see www.copgtp.org for more information. Bob Knight and colleagues in 2009 summarised the competences and knowledge base that practitioners require for working with older people. Their paper has become known as the Pike's Peak model for training since the group met to discuss these competencies in the valley below Pike's Peak in Colorado. Four broad areas of professional practice define the work of professionals specialising in work with older people. These revolve around knowledge about lifespan development, psychopathology in later life, understanding comorbid chronic medical conditions as presenting features in work with older people, and appreciating the diversity of the range of age-specific environmental contexts when working with older people. Laidlaw and Pachana (2009) (later republished in 2011 in the APA *Monitor* as continuing education credit) provide an international perspective on the implications of demographic change for psychologists working with older people, whereas Karel et al. (2012) review the professional implications of demographic trends from a more US-centric perspective.

Summary

CBT is a challenging and demanding form of psychotherapy as it entails learning a set of techniques and procedures and following a model for structuring sessions. It may not be easy to 'pick up and play', but this is sometimes the message novice therapists can be given when it comes to CBT. It requires discipline and training to become adept at CBT and in reality it takes years to become skilled. Even then the effectiveness of CBT therapists may be diminished if they do not continue with appropriate CPD and make time for regular professional peer supervision. At the same time, the basic idea of CBT is simple and elegant. It has a set of ideas and an approach that patients easily and quickly understand will be helpful for them in better managing their problems. As such, time invested in learning CBT is time well spent, and using this book is one part of your professional development.

Learning Log: Reflection and Review
What have you gained from reading over this first chapter?

- Think about the cognitive model for depression and anxiety, and in particular think about how it may apply with your clients. Does the overt and covert distinction offer any advantages to the way you may conceptualise their presentation?

- Can you chart a course for yourself to become more specialised in working with older people? Perhaps you need to attend some specialist workshops or advanced training. Can you identify a supervisor with an interest/specialist skills in working with this client group? Can you identify what steps you may wish to take along your route to become more skilled with this client group? Perhaps you can create a diagram/chart for you to record your progress.
- Consider clients you have worked with before. Consider what characteristics and presenting problems you can recall from the start of therapy. Did these characteristics and presenting problems fill you with optimism or pessimism about the possibilities for change? What are the suitable criteria for CBT that you can discern?
- Consider what the difference between augmenting and adapting therapy would make to your own clinical practice. This may be especially important for clients for which there is a less well-developed evidence base, e.g. CBT for depression/anxiety in dementia.

Further Reading

The following sources provide more in-depth coverage of the topics raised in this chapter.

Beck, A. T., Rush, A. J., Shaw, B. F., & Emery, G. (1979). *Cognitive therapy of depression*. New York: Guilford Press.

Mueller, M., Kennerley, H., McManus, F., & Westbrook, D. (2010). *The Oxford guide to surviving as a CBT therapist*. Oxford: Oxford University Press.

Westbrook, D., Kennerley, H., & Kirk, J. (2011). *An introduction to cognitive behaviour therapy: skills and application* (2nd ed.). London: SAGE.

Two

Practical Information for Psychotherapists Working with Older People

Learning Objectives
By the end of this chapter you will:

- Understand what demographic change is and the implications for therapists working with older people
- Understand about the experiences of ageing and the development of new cohorts of older people
- Understand that attitudes to ageing can be influenced by depression and anxiety and may act as pre-existing vulnerabilities for individuals who internalise negative age stereotypes

Introduction

In this chapter, it helps to understand that there are general facts and individual experiences about working with older clients. It is important to reconcile the two while differentiating one from the other. It may seem as if there is too much external information you need to equip yourself with *prior* to working with older people. In reality that is not the case.

> While there may be new issues to consider when working with older people, skills learned in therapy with other populations (e.g. adults) can translate well to older people.

The first thing you need to work successfully with older people is the same thing you need to work successfully with any client, and that is to develop a curiosity towards understanding the individual as fully as possible, with an openness to being collaborative and an expectation for optimal functioning from the outset. It may be useful for you to consider what your beliefs about ageing are prior to working with older people. Perhaps you might want to take this 'pop quiz' before you read any further? (The answers are at the end of the chapter).

What Do You Know About Ageing and Mental Health? Test Yourself

1. In the UK life expectancy at birth (females) is now:
   A. 70   B. 82   C. 62   D. 90

2. What is the life expectancy for women aged 65 years, i.e. if you reach 65 how much longer can you expect to live?
   A. 5 years   B. 10 years   C. 20 years   D. 25 years

3. The number of centenarians has increased dramatically over the last century. At the turn of the last century (1900) there were approximately 100 centenarians alive in the UK. How many centenarians are alive in the UK today?
   A. 1,000   B. 2,500   C. 8,000   D. 12,500

4. Older people outnumber younger people in the UK:
   A. True   B. False

5. The fastest-growing section of society is people aged 60–70:
   A. True   B. False

6. Depression in later life is very common and the prevalence increases as people get older:
   A. True   B. False

7. Depression is an understandable reaction to the challenges of growing older as loss accumulates as people age:
   A. True   B. False

8. Anxiety is more common than depression in later life:
   A. True   B. False

9. Dementia is an outcome of old age:
   A. True   B. False

10. How many people live with dementia in the UK (the current UK population is 63 million[1])?
    A. 800,000   B. 1 million   C. 3 million   D. 8 million

---

[1] UK population based on data from the Office for National Statistics website www.ons.gov.uk/ons/taxonomy/index.html?nsci=Population (accessed 28 December 2012).

Demographic Change and the New Cohort of Older People

People are living longer than any previous generations. In transit through an airport recently I was struck by an arresting advertising billboard: 'Two-thirds of the people who have ever reached 65 are alive today' (www.hsbcusa.com/ourcompany/pressroom/2010/news_09302010_newyork_discover.html). The growth in numbers of people living longer is testified by the fact that two people celebrate their 60th birthday every second around the world (UNFPA, 2012). Longevity being achieved by people now in the developed and developing world are unprecedented in the whole of human history (Kinsella & Wan, 2009; UN, 2011), and with morbidity compressed to the last stage of life (Fries, 2003) there is much to be optimistic about.

> Ageing is a process rather than a state. Chronological age is often the least useful thing to know about a person. Most people think of themselves as younger than their chronological age.
> Being older is just another stage of life. It is not necessarily something to be endured.

Healthy life expectancy (HLE) is the number of years an individual may expect to live in good or very good health, whereas, *disability-free life expectancy* (DFLE) is the number of years an individual may expect to live free from a chronic and limiting illness or disability (ONS, 2011c).

> Current life expectancy at age 65 years for men and women in the UK is 18 and 20 years respectively.

At birth and at age 65, HLE & DFLE is higher for women than men. However, men spend lower proportions of their lives in illness or disability compared to women. At age 65 in the UK, men can expect to live in very good or good health (HLE) for 10 years whereas women at age 65 can expect to live for 11.5 years. At the same age, but considering DFLE, men can expect to live for 10 years and women can expect to live for 11 years free from a limiting chronic illness or disability (ONS, 2011c).

In 1900, average life expectancy in the developed world was 45 to 50 years. Now, life expectancy at birth in the developed world is currently 78 years, but by 2050 life expectancy at birth will be 83 years (UNFPA, 2012).

> Many of the current cohort of older people are going to live beyond their own expectations for lifespan and beyond that of their own parents and grandparents.

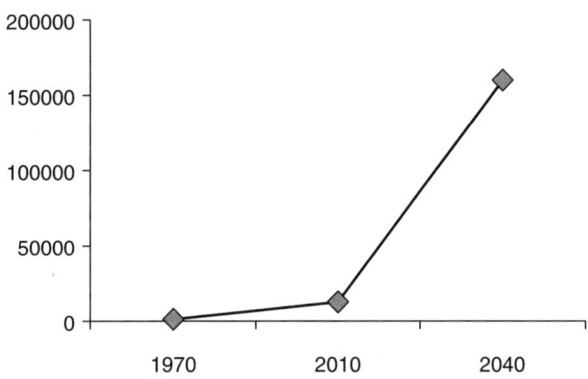

Centenarians Alive in the UK

FIGURE 2.1 *Exponential increase in number of people aged 100 alive in the UK from 1970 to 2040 (ONS, 2011a)*

In the UK, life expectancy at birth has reached its highest ever level in the UK, with a life expectancy of 82 years for a female born today and 78 years for a male born today (ONS, 2011a). Ageing is a gender issue, with greater numbers of older women than men alive. As people age the ratio of women to men increases with the effect that men and women experience ageing differently. Older men are more likely to be living with their spouse whereas older women are more likely to be widowed and living on their own (Laidlaw & Pachana, 2011).

The oldest-old section of society is increasing the fastest. In the UK in 1970 there were 1,180 centenarians alive, whereas this figure increased almost 12-fold to 12,640 in 2010 (ONS, 2011a). By mid-2040 (see Figure 2.1), according to UK population projections, the number of centenarians alive in the UK is estimated to reach 160,000 persons, a more than 12-fold increase over 2010 figures (ONS, 2011b).

The 'new cohort' of older people are likely to have more complex family and intergenerational structures, may be more likely to have increased take up of other medical services due to multiple comorbidities due to increased longevity, and a subgroup may also have greater levels of psychiatric complexity. In Europe and North America, life expectancy at birth from 1950 to 2100 increased from age 66–87 years for Europe and 69–88 years for North America as a whole (UN, 2011). Life expectancy at age 75 has also increased, with an average life expectancy of between 11 and 12 years in the UK and USA (UN, 2011).

Linked to increases in longevity is a decline in fertility, thus in the developed world many societies have larger populations aged 60-plus in comparison to those aged 15 years and under.

Ageing in the UK

In comparison to other European countries the UK is ageing more gradually and by 2035 will have one of the lowest proportions of its population aged 65 years plus

(ONS, 2012). For a more in-depth comparison of the UK ageing profile with that of other European countries the reader is directed to the DEMOS (2012) report. In 2010, 17 per cent of the population was aged 65 years and older, but by 2035 it is expected that this figure will increase to 23 per cent (see Figure 2.2). Over the same period, the population aged 16 years and under will decrease from 19 per cent to 18 per cent. By 2035 the population described as the oldest-old (those aged 85 and above) will increase by more than 60 per cent from 1.4 million in 2010 to 3.6 million in 2035, accounting for 5 per cent of the total UK population (ONS, 2011c).

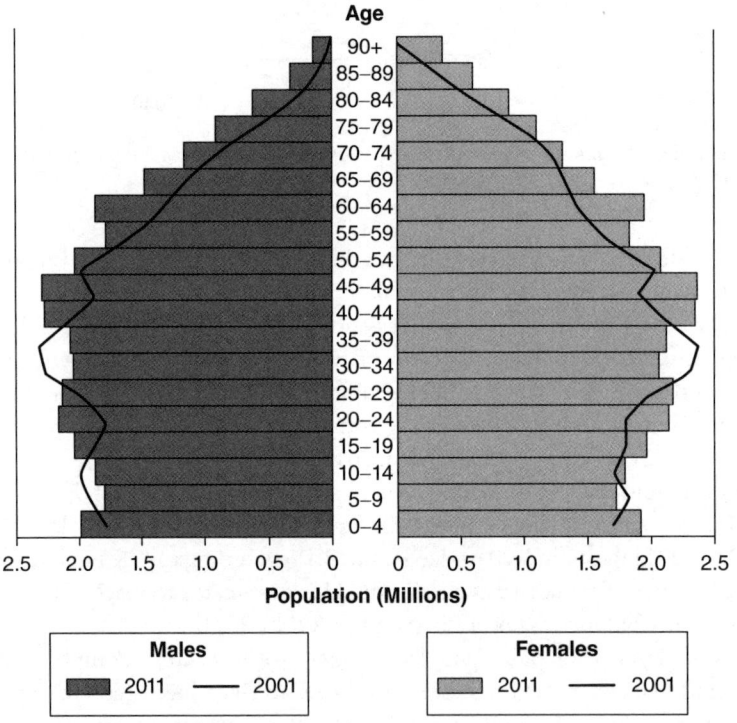

FIGURE 2.2   *Population pyramid for the UK 2001–2011*

Source: ONS (2012)

Working with Older People: Positive Exemplars of Ageing

For those who wish to work most effectively with older people, there needs to be an openness to the possibility for change and growth at all ages. It is important to try and challenge our expectations for ageing and older people in as many ways as we can. In Figure 2.3 there are a couple of exemplars of 'super agers' – people who continue to grow and thrive throughout their lives.

Regrettably, the negative stereotypical image of ageing as being about loss and decrepitude still holds enormous power for older people themselves (Bodner, 2009)

Positive exemplars of ageing:	
Hedda Bolger is 102 years old and still working as a psychotherapist in Los Angeles, CA. She has featured in a documentary on ageing (see www.beautyofageing.com). She was awarded an outstanding worker award at a ceremony in Washington DC. She is still pursuing her goals and is still active. She considers this stage of life to be a good one. She continues to remain invested in planning for the future.	Fauja Singh was born in India in 1911. He moved to London to be with his son, after his wife died. To pass the time, Fauja Singh started running marathons at the age of 89. He has set records for the fastest time of 80 and 90 years old marathon runners. At over 100 years he continued to run marathons. In April 2012 he ran the London Marathon in under 8 hours at the age of 101. He stopped competitive racing at the age of 102, after completing a 10km race in Hong Kong in February 2013 in which he had improved on his time for the race a year previously.
Pause for thought: What are your thoughts about these individuals? What does it tell you about how people are ageing:	

FIGURE 2.3   *Positive exemplars of ageing*

and even for therapists. However, rates of depression and anxiety in later life may actually be lower than rates reported for younger or middle-aged adults (Blazer, 2010). When working with depressed or anxious older people, or when working with people with dementia, it may be useful for clinicians to remember that the majority of older people age successfully. Furthermore, Carstensen et al. (2011), in their longitudinal follow-up of a cohort of adults ranging in age from 18 to 94 over 10 years, demonstrate that emotional stability and well-being improves with age.

Perhaps you can take a moment to reflect on what you have learned about ageing and changing demographics before you read on further. You might want to use Table 2.1 to note some thoughts on your reflections.

TABLE 2.1   *Reflection on ageing*

Reflection point: what are your thoughts about growing older? How does this information impact on them?	
Positive aspects of ageing	Negative aspects, or your fears about these
How do the columns balance out? Is there action for you to take? Make a specific plan for yourself to address any fears, or make a plan to read further in terms of interests piqued by this section.	

A copy of this table is available to download from https://study.sagepub.com/laidlaw

> ### Key Messages About Demographic Change
> - People are living longer and healthier than at any time in human history
> - The oldest-old subset of the population is growing the fastest, thus there are likely to be many more older people in their eighth and ninth decade who may present for therapy
> - The number of people with dementia is set to increase, and with diagnosis being made at an earlier stage there may be a demand for psychological therapy to help people manage the transition this diagnosis entails
> - The 'baby boomers' are about to become the new cohort of older people and as this generation is noted for its non-conformity in the past there are expectations that they will create a new way to be old
> - People in their 60s and 70s rarely consider themselves old and therapists need to watch out for their own implicit ageist attitudes

When Does Someone Become Old?

Ageing is a *process* rather than a state, with a great deal of heterogeneity in how people experience ageing. Growing old doesn't need to be equated with becoming decrepit, as ageing is a unique experience determined by a number of factors such as contact with positive role models, societal attitudes and norms, and a person's idiosyncratic appraisals of events and physical or emotional changes.

Diehl and Werner-Wahl (2010) propose that the subjective nature of an individual's experience of ageing can be understood by reference to the concept of awareness of age-related change (AARC; Diehl & Werner-Wahl, 2010), with understanding occurring along multidimensional perspectives and experiences. A person only becomes subjectively aware of their personal experience of ageing by perceiving that life may have changed due to some consequence of ageing. These may be intrapersonal and interpersonal consequences and have behavioural, cognitive or affective outcomes for the individual.

In the model proposed by Diehl and Werner-Wahl (2010), awareness may not be entirely internalised, but could be as a result of external consequences of ageing coming within the focal awareness of the individual such as prejudice or discrimination. Central to understanding the experience of ageing is that changes are attributed to age and are perceived as either positive or negative (expressly not neutral). The subjective AARC may not necessarily align with objective change. It is the individual's attribution of the impact of events that is more important in determining a sense of becoming older. AARC very clearly places the individual as being responsive to their internal and external environments, and explains how it is that chronological age is not the primary factor that people draw upon when becoming aware of being 'old'.

There is a great deal of heterogeneity in the population grouping of older people, with up to four generations contained therein. A person in their 60s is often very different to a person in their 90s, but both may be considered elderly people. Most people in their 60s do not consider themselves old, and as people live longer we may need to revise our age definitions. Currently the UN defines old age as starting at 60 (UNFPA, 2012). Typically, people can be classified as young-old, old-old, and sometimes also oldest-old. The age definitions for this vary, but originated from the noted gerontologist Bernice Neugarten (Neugarten et al., 1961) who classified the young-old as people aged between 65 and 74 years and the oldest-old as aged 76 years and above. Baltes and Smith (2003) use the descriptors third age (approximately 65–80 years) and fourth age (80 or 85 years plus) to differentiate the ageing experience of young-old and old-old people. The fourth age is when the greatest challenges associated with ageing may be experienced.

Demographic Change and Implications for Therapists

As a consequence of demographic change, many more psychotherapists are increasingly likely to come into contact with older people seeking help, and in all probability the issues older people bring into therapy will change as the person experiences ageing (Karel et al., 2012; Laidlaw & Pachana, 2011). Therapists may be ill-prepared to meet the needs of older people in therapy, and therefore moves towards outlining specific skills and competences that therapists may wish to consider when working with older people are being developed (Knight et al., 2009). If psychological therapists wish to meet the needs of their older clients, they will need to invest in the development of their competencies in geropsychology practice (see Karel et al., 2012).

Negative Attitudes to Ageing and Clinical Outcome

Older people without physical or psychological problems report positive attitudes to ageing (Bryant et al., 2012; Quinn et al., 2009; Shenkin et al., 2014). However, older people can be quite ageist (a term coined by Robert Butler, see Achenbaum, 2013) – they sometimes hold on to negative stereotypical and discriminatory beliefs about ageing (Bodner, 2009). Thus, when asked about oneself, an older person may not see themselves as different from the adult working age population, but may consider the group of older people in more negative ways (Johnson, 2013). Thus one should not be surprised if older people appear to hold ageist views and beliefs. This could become an important focus for psychoeducation in CBT in early sessions. The AAQ (Laidlaw et al., 2004) is a 24-item self-report cross-cultural scale that may help you assess whether your client has a negative attitude to ageing as it contains both negative and positive experiences of ageing. Developed in 19 countries with a field-trial sample of 5,566 participants the scale is free to use.

When a person is depressed or anxious this may influence the perceptions, expectations and consequently the behaviour of an individual (Chachamovich et al., 2008). Research suggests that attitudes to ageing may be mood-state dependent, and rather than being fixed and unchangeable negative attitudes to ageing are determined by elevation in an individual's scores on depression scales (Chachamovich et al., 2008; Shenkin et al., 2014). Attitudes to ageing may also be determined by prior experience of mental illness – as Quinn et al. (2009) note, older people with a history of contact with psychiatric services have more negative attitudes to ageing. Those participants with a more positive attitude to ageing engaged in more healthy behaviours and higher rates of well-being, giving clinicians food for thought when working with depressed or anxious older people.

Therapists working with older people may need to be aware that an older person does not necessarily identify with their 'in-group' (i.e. other older people) and in all likelihood will not see themselves as old – they therefore may be offended if you refer to them as old or elderly. Depressed older people may have attitudes to ageing that act as a negative filter, and they may be more inclined to see the future as something to be dreaded. Therapists need to bear in mind that this is mood-state dependent and is not necessarily a statement of fact. Once the depression has resolved people will be less pessimistic about the future and less concerned with age.

Summary

People are living longer, are generally happier in later life (Frijters & Beatton, 2012), and are living generally healthier lives with evidence of compression of morbidity to later stages of life (Fries, 2003). The majority of older people do not develop depression or anxiety, and easily accommodate the transition into later life. Thus, when working clinically with older people there may be a need for clinicians to question their own attitudes to ageing and understandings as these may be biased and influenced because of contact with distressed older people who may not represent the norm for ageing.

Learning Log: Reflection and Review
What have you gained from reading over this chapter?

- Think about the impact of the global demographic transition and increasing longevity. How might it change the type of clients you may work with in the future. Does the change in demographics seem to be reflected in your caseload or in the types of referrals your service receives? If not, why might this be?
- Have you been surprised by any of the information on the demographics of ageing presented in this chapter? What has been the most surprising fact you have learned and what made this so surprising to you?
- Can you think of a case you worked with recently where you may have been tempted to believe that their problems are 'understandable' because of life-span experiences or because your client convinced you that age was the main reason for their problems?
- When you think about older people you may know personally, what seems to be their experience of ageing? Do they fit the stereotype of frail, confused vulnerable people or are they different?

Further Reading

The following sources provide more in-depth coverage of topics raised in this chapter.

Kinsella, K. & Wan, H. (2009). *US Census Bureau, series P95/09–1, an ageing world: 2008*, Washington, DC: US Government Printing Office. Available at: www.census.gov/prod/2009pubs/p95–09–1.pdf

UNFPA, United Nations Population Fund and HelpAge International (2012). *Ageing in the twenty-first century: a celebration and a challenge*. New York: UNFPA.

You may want to consult AGE UK's 2012–2013 series on improving later life. These are a series of booklets written in non-scientific language that debunk myths of ageing. They are available free to download at: www.ageuk.org.uk/professional-resources-home/knowledge-hub-evidence-statistics/improving-later-life-series

Answers to Pop Quiz

Well, here are the answers. Checkout how much you already know.

1. In the UK life expectancy at birth (females) is now:
   A. 70   B. 82   C 62   D. 90

   Answer is B. According to the Office of National Statistics (ONS, 2011a) the UK has reached its highest ever level for life expectancy at birth.

2. What is the life expectancy for women aged 65 years, i.e. if you reach 65 how much longer can you expect to live?
   A. 5 years   B. 10 years   C. 20 years   D. 25 years.

   Answer is C. According to the Office of National Statistics (www.ons.gov.uk/ons/rel/lifetables/interim-life-tables/2008-2010/sum-ilt-2008-10.html accessed May 2012), life expectancy at age 65 in the UK is 20.4 years at age 65 for females and 17.8 years for men.

3. The number of centenarians has increased dramatically over the last century. At the turn of the last century (1900) there were approximately 100 centenarians alive in the UK. How many centenarians are alive in the UK today?
   A. 1,000   B. 2,500   C. 8,000   D. 12,500

   Answer is D. According to the Office of National Statistics (ONS, 2011a), there were 12,640 centenarians alive in the UK in 2010.

4. Older people outnumber younger people in the UK:
   A. True   B. False

   Answer is True. Since 2007 (ONS, 2011b) there are more people entitled to state pensions than people aged under 16.

5. The fastest-growing section of society is people aged 60–70:
   A. True   B. False

   Answer is False. The UN (2011) note that global population totals of people aged 80 plus will increase by a factor of 8, whereas the population aged 60 plus will triple between now and 2100.

6. Depression in later life is very common and the prevalence increases as people get older:
   A. True   B. False

   Answer is False. The prevalence of depression is lower in older adults compared to adults of working and does not necessarily increase exponentially as one ages.

7. Depression is an understandable reaction to the challenges of growing older as loss accumulates as people age:
   A. True   B. False

   Answer is False. Rates of depression are surprisingly uncommon when considering the challenges that can be posed by old age (Sadavoy, 2009).

8. Anxiety is more common than depression in later life:
   A. True   B. False

   Answer is True. Anxiety is more common than depression, but it remains under-recognised and undertreated in primary care in terms of its impact on well-being and as a risk factor for disability and death (Bryant et al., 2008).

9. Dementia is an outcome of old age:
   A. True   B. False

   Answer is False. Alzheimer's disease is more common in older people and rates of Alzheimer's disease do certainly increase with age. This does not mean that dementia is an outcome of old age as we would be seeing at least the majority of the very oldest people developing dementia, whereas the minority develop it.

10. How many people live with dementia in the UK?
    A. 800,000   B. 1 million   C. 3 million   D. 8 million

    Answer is A. Currently in the UK, according to the recent Dementia 2010 report (www.dementia2010.org/), an estimated 821,884 people live with dementia and it is projected to increase to 1 million people by 2025.

Three
CBT for Late Life Depression

Learning Objectives

By the end of this chapter you will:

- Learn about the prevalence of depression in later life
- Become knowledgeable about measurement issues in late depression
- Be able to select the most appropriate assessment measure for depression in terms of diagnostic value, symptom severity and utility as a measure of change
- Understand the efficacy data for CBT for depression in later life

Depression in Later Life

Depression and anxiety are major causes of mental health problems in later life, but rates of major depressive disorder are lower in older people compared to younger or middle-aged adults (Blazer, 2010; Blazer & Hybels, 2005; Jorm, 2000). Beekman et al. (1999) calculate a prevalence rate of 13.5 per cent for clinically relevant depression symptoms.

> Rates of depression are surprisingly uncommon when considering the challenges that can be posed by old age (Sadavoy, 2009) and the prevalence of depression is lower in older adults compared to adults of working age (Jorm, 2000).

Using a subset of a large sample, McDougall et al. (2007) reported findings from a large epidemiological study looking at the prevalence of depression in people aged 65 years and older from across England and Wales. They estimated the prevalence of depression among older people to be 8.7 per cent, with a prevalence rate for severe depression of 2.7 per cent. There did not appear to be a relationship between age and prevalence of depression, but factors associated with increased risk for depression were: being female, experiencing medical comorbidity, disability, and social deprivation.

'Given the plethora of risk for late life depression, we find it easy to focus upon these risks. Yet a balanced perspective will augment our ability to treat our patients effectively . . . Many times, we find ourselves surprised when one of our older patients adapts to a stressor more effectively than we could ever imagine' (Blazer, 2010: 172).

However, subsyndromal or 'subclinical' depression (subclinical depression is the presence of significant symptoms of depression that don't fully meet diagnostic criteria for major depression) appears to be much more common in older people (Alexopoulous, 2005). Subsyndromal depression often develops into a chronic condition as the naturalistic outcome is poor, with a strong association of increased mortality in older people with subclinical depression (Lyness, 2008).

Depression is *not* an outcome of old age. People may become depressed for a whole host of reasons. Losses and challenges associated with ageing may in some instances be a contributory factor for some people, but it is more likely to be the idiosyncratic way a person makes sense of things that determines the personal impact of a situation. Be sure to understand the meaning and personal relevance of a situation rather than assuming it is a feature of ageing.

Clinicians inexperienced in working with older people often overestimate the prevalence of depression and underestimate the possibility of good treatment outcomes, as depression is seen as 'justifiable' and 'understandable' (Burroughs et al., 2006). There may be a mistaken belief that depression in later life results from the 'fallacy of good reasons' (Unutzer et al., 1999: 235) where providers attribute the onset and maintenance of problems to 'old age' and believe there is no point in intervening, as they erroneously believe problems to be unchangeable.

Jorm (2000) notes that when studies assess age differences in depression and anxiety, and systematically control for risk factors, depression is shown to reduce with age. Blazer (2010) explains the paradox of low relative rates of depression in the presence of challenges associated with ageing in terms of three protective factors such as: (i) mature emotional regulation competence, consistent with the work by Carstensen's theory of socio-emotional selectivity theory (Carstensen et al., 1999); (ii) increased wisdom (Baltes & Smith, 2008) due to managing life experiences; and (iii) resilience, as older people cope better with stressful events (see Chapter 4 for more on this issue).

Blazer (2010: 172) notes that events experienced as being 'on time', such as bereavements, may be anticipated and accepted by older people as being a fact of life, therefore promoting better coping with these events. Echoing this, Sadavoy (2009) notes that rates of depression are surprisingly uncommon considering the challenges that can be posed by old age. Consistent with this evidence, and contrary to the notion that old age is a stage of life to be feared, is the ageing paradox where older people typically report high levels of life satisfaction at the stage of life most associated with cognitive and physical decline (Carstensen & Lockerhoff, 2003).

Assessment and Measurement of Mental Health in Later Life

The development of robust and effective assessment tools is a complex issue. When choosing a measurement tool to use, the clinician needs to exercise judgement in how a tool may be used and to serve what purpose.

When using any assessment tool, one must consider issues of validity (i.e. a tool should measure what it is intended to) and reliability (i.e. the consistency and stability of the reported scores from a tool by the same person on more than one occasion), as well as how well a tool performs in terms of specificity (i.e. measures depression as opposed to anxiety) and sensitivity (i.e. it is adequate for detecting depression when it exists). Measurement is very important, and clinicians must consider scores in light of other factors. When considering the choice and use of measurement tools with older people, clinicians must also assess whether the tool they wish to use has been validated with older people. Additionally, a practical consideration may be whether the measurement tool is free or costs money. The service needs may also determine the choice of measurement tool, and sometimes a minimum data set is agreed that is adopted from adult services.

The Royal College of Psychiatrists' Faculty of the Psychiatry of Old Age produced a useful assessment guideline for individual patient outcome measurement. The RCP document (2012) reminds us that one should not assess only mental health indices but also take account of quality of life and other social outcomes.

For assessment of depression, the RCP recommend the Geriatric Depression Scale (GDS) in its 30-item, 15-item and 10-item formats. In the same report, the Hospital Anxiety and Depression Scale (HADS) and the Patient Health Questionnaire (PHQ-9) are both recommended for use with older people. For situations where a person is diagnosed with dementia, to assess for depression the RCP (2012) recommend the use of the Cornell Scale for Depression in Dementia (CSDD). This last measure developed by Alexopoulos et al. (1988) is a 19-item observer-rated measure, based around five domains (mood-related signs, behavioural disturbance, physical signs, cyclic (diurnal) variance, and ideational disturbance). It is administered by interview with a family 'informant' of the person with dementia, as well as a direct observation and interview with the individual to determine if depression is present. Scores above 8 suggest that significant depression symptoms may be present, whereas a score above 12 indicates probable depression. Although the CSDD is quite simple it can take quite a degree of skill on the part of the interviewer to extract relevant and appropriate information to make an accurate evaluation of mood disorder in someone with dementia.

Assessment Tools with Older People with Depression

When considering how useful a measure may be you ought to consider four factors:

- *Validity* – does it measure what it says it does?
- *Reliability* – can you trust this measure to be accurate and to do so at different times, i.e. will you get the same scores under the same condition consistently?
- *Sensitivity* – does it measure things at a level you'd expect without being set too low (over diagnosing) or too high (underdiagnosing)?
- *Specificity* – does it measure the one main condition and not a whole mix of conditions, i.e. if it is a depression scale does it measure depression and allow you to differentiate these symptoms from anxiety symptoms?

While the Beck Depression Inventory (BDI) and the PHQ-9 are reliable and valid in assessing depression in older people, there is no one particular 'gold standard' measure designed to be used with older people other than perhaps the GDS (Yesavage et al., 1983). As with any measure, the GDS is not without its flaws. Nonetheless, used prudently it can be very useful in assessment with older people. It is free, simple to use, quick to administer and provides clear cut-off scores. The other main advantage of the GDS is that it avoids the use of somatic items that can potentially inflate scores with older people (Yesavage et al., 1983; Wancata et al., 2006).

The Geriatric Depression Scales (GDS; Yesavage et al., 1983)

The original GDS was a 30-item self-report scale with a simple yes–no answer format. It was designed to be used with older people and to differentiate physical from psychological symptoms of depression. In the main the most commonly used versions of the GDS would appear to be the original GDS-30 and the original short-form GDS-15. There are so many different formats for the GDS from the original long form (30 item; Yesavage et al., 1983), with numerous different language versions supported by a website (www.stanford.edu/~yesavage/GDS.html) that provides a forum for disseminating and distributing different versions. Wancata et al. (2006) note that the most frequently used cut-off score for the GDS-30 is 10 or 11. For the GDS-15, the most frequently used cut-off score is 5 or 6. In reviewing their evidence, Wancata et al. (2006) confirm that the GDS is *not* a sensitive tool for detecting depression in people with dementia.

Dennis et al. (2012) reviewed a number of screening tools for the detection of depression in acutely ill hospitalised older people, and reported that the GDS-15 and the GDS-30 are the most systematically evaluated tools for this population and this setting. The GDS has been used successfully with people exhibiting mild cognitive impairment (Debruyne et al., 2009), and as a screen for depression after stroke (Cinamon et al., 2010; Sivrioglu et al., 2009) and depression in Parkinson's disease

(Ertan et al., 2005).When using this scale for detecting depression in Parkinson's disease, Ertan et al. (2005) suggest that a cut-off score of 13/14 gives the optimal values of specificity and sensitivity.

Perhaps the most commonly used version of the GDS is the original short form, the GDS-15, although the RCP (2012) also recommend the use of the GDS-10 (D'Ath et al., 1994; Shah et al., 1997). Nonetheless, Mitchell et al. (2010) recommend the use of the GDS-15 over the GDS-30. In a recent review, Mitchell et al. (2010) suggest that the original version GDS-15 performs better than the long form of the GDS (GDS-30) in primary care settings.

As brevity of assessment is a very useful feature in clinical settings, and researchers have developed short forms of the GDS over the years that are even briefer. The GDS-5 (Rinaldi et al., 2003) and GDS-4 (Shah et al., 1997) have become available and claim to match the sensitivity and specificity of the GDS-15 in the detection of depression.These very short scales are less likely to function as sensitive measures for change in symptom profile, and in therapy the shorter versions of the GDS may not be as useful for indicating areas for intervention. Izal et al. (2010) note that a problem with many of the new versions of the short GDS scales are that they are derived from the GDS-15 and will therefore tend to share their flaws. Izal and colleagues have derived a new form of the GDS-10 they call the GDS-R, with items for this scale drawn from the GDS-30. The GDS-R is different from the GDS-10 (Shah et al., 1997) and the optimal cut-off score is 5 (3 for the GDS-10) with very high levels of sensitivity and specificity.Thus, the process for choosing to use the GDS is becoming increasingly complex. For quick screening the GDS-5 may suffice, whereas the GDS-10 or GDS-R may be better but still retain brevity. For measurement purposes over time the GDS-15 may be optimal.

The Hospital Anxiety and Depression Scale (HADS; Zigmond & Snaith, 1983)

The HADS used to be a freely available measure but must now be purchased and used under licence. It is a 14-item self-report scale with seven items purported to measure anxiety symptoms and seven items purported to measure depression symptoms. It is very useful as it was designed to detect depression and anxiety in medically ill patients, hence with older people with chronic physical illnesses it may be a useful measure to detect emotional distress and to avoid inflated scores due to the influence of medical complaints. Bjelland et al. (2002) reviewed the data reported for the use of the HADS and confirmed a two-factor structure (anxiety and depression) for this scale, as well as confirming optimal sensitivity and specificity for a cut-off score of 8+ for anxiety and depression with this measure. Concurrent validity of this measure with other scales measuring depression and anxiety (separately) were good. Moderate to high correlations[1] between the anxiety and depression domains of this scale suggests each domain

---

[1] A correlation is a relationship between variables. Usually one reports correlation coefficients, which is a means of assessing the strength of a relationship between variables with a correlation coefficient closer to 1 being strongest. Correlation does not imply causation.

may in fact be measuring the same construct, and that remains a big question-mark over the utility of this measure. Norton et al. (2013) recommend that as the HADS does not provide adequate separation between the anxiety and depression subscales, it should be used as a more general measure of distress. Thus clinicians are advised to exercise caution in their use of this measure and consider carefully whether it may be more efficient to assess anxiety and depression separately.

The Beck Depression Inventory (BDI; Beck et al., 1996)

The BDI is a very well known self-report measure of depression consisting of 21 items linked to DSM-IV (APA, 2000) diagnostic criteria. Of course the DSM-5 is now updating a number of aspects of the DSM-IV (see APA, 2013), but much of the published research studies use DSM-IV.

The BDI is not a diagnostic tool per se, more a measure of symptom severity, and as such can be a very useful measure of symptom change when carrying out a treatment evaluation. It needs to be purchased and used under licence. The BDI-II can be criticised for having somatic scale items – this may inflate scores when used with older people, and therefore caution is advised. The BDI-II uses a more complex response scale for people to self-rate their symptoms of depression and therefore may not be appropriate to use with older people with cognitive impairment (Edelstein et al., 2008). Nevertheless, the BDI-II has been a staple of many outcome trials evaluating CBT in later life. Segal et al. (2008) provide the most comprehensive evaluation of the psychometric properties of the BDI-II with older people, and as one might expect there are no differences in cut-offs between younger and older people with good reliability and validity data with older people (Segal et al., 2008).

The Patient Health Questionnaire (PHQ-9; Spitzer et al., 1999)

This measure is used for evaluating outcome (as it is sensitive to change) as part of the IAPT initiative in the UK, and is also commonly used by GPs in primary care. The PHQ-9 is a simple 9-item scale originally derived from a larger 60-item scale. It is scored from 0 to 3 for each item, so that a maximum score of 27 is rated as severe depression, with a score of 4 or less indicating no symptoms of depression. A score of 15 or more on this measure is considered a 'red flag', indicating a score that suggests treatment is warranted. The PHQ-9 is based on the DSM-IV primary diagnostic criteria for major depressive disorder, so this scale can be used diagnostically (Kroenke & Spitzer, 2002), and for brief assessments a PHQ-2 based on the first two questions of the full scale is also available. The cut-off scores for the PHQ-9 are as follows: 5–9 indicates mild depression, 10–14 is moderate depression, 15–19 is moderately severe, and 20 plus is severe (Kroenke & Spitzer, 2002). The PHQ-9 is freely available on www.phqscreeners.com.

The PHQ-9 has been used with older people and is recommended for use by the RCP (2012). Lowe et al. (2004), using data from the IMPACT (Improving Mood-Promoting Access to Collaborative Treatment) trial, confirmed the superiority of the

PHQ-9 as a diagnostic tool for detecting depression, but also demonstrated that the PHQ-9 was a reliable measure of treatment outcome with older people.

The PHQ-9 has further demonstrated its utility with older people. Ell et al. (2005) show that it functions well as a screen for depression in older people living in care homes. Williams et al. (2005) note that the PHQ-9 works well as a screening tool for depression in older people who have had a stroke. A cut-off score of 10 on this tool provided an optimal score for sensitivity and specificity purposes. The PHQ-9 successfully classified depressed from non-depressed individuals with a stroke. For such a brief measure this is very useful, especially as the data reported by Williams et al. (2005) suggest the PHQ-9 scores are invariant with regard to age, ethnicity and gender.

Other scales such as CES-D (Haringsma et al., 2004), CORE-OM (Barkham et al., 2005) and DASS (Gloster et al., 2008) have also been evaluated for use with older people with some support, although these measures are less commonly used. For further information readers can consult a very thorough review of the use of standardised measures with older people by Edelstein et al. (2008).

> ## Empirical Evidence of CBT for Depression with Older People: Becoming a Sophisticated Consumer of Research
>
> - Prevalence of depression is lower in older people in comparison to that for adults of working age.
> - Depression is higher in conditions where there is medical comorbidity, and is particularly elevated following a stroke or in conditions such as dementia and Parkinson's disease. There is good evidence that depression in these conditions is amenable to treatment using psychological therapy such as CBT.
> - Depression is sometimes erroneously construed as an 'understandable' reaction to the losses and challenges of ageing, but the majority of older people do not develop depression.
> - Depression may be more likely to be subclinical than major depressive disorders.
> - There is a range of psychometrically robust assessment tools for use with older people, with the GDS-15 and PHQ-9 being particularly recommended in primary care settings.

PRISMA is Preferred Reporting Items for Systematic Reviews (SR) and Meta-Analyses (MA), producing an evidence-based set of criteria for evaluating SRs and MAs (Moher et al., 2009). PRISMA facilitates the critical evaluation of systematic reviews and helps ensure reported bias is kept to a minimum, but this cannot be eradicated completely (Moher et al., 2009).

Some reviews are completed by researchers without any experience of conducting randomised controlled trials, with evident lack of clinical insights. There are pros and cons of this as some reviewers who have completed clinical trials are inadvertently partisan in approach. Reading research presented in systematic reviews requires the reader to adopt a critically evaluative stance, as despite the advent of guides such as Cochrane Review Guidelines and PRISMA criteria, there is still work required by the reader. A recent book by Scogin and Shah (2012) provides a comprehensive guide to evidence-based psychological treatments with older people and may be a useful additional reading source for those who wish to investigate the evidence base in more detail. The data in tables over the next few pages show how difficult it is to determine the evidence from looking at systematic reviews, and these reviews are inevitably subject to a form of internal error as reviewers make decisions on data reported in brief peer-reviewed publications. Thus, when publishing data there is limited space to give a full account of complicated randomisation procedures and other methodological aspects.[2] Some reviews also characterise a control condition, such as *treatment as usual* (TAU), as a passive control condition. TAU, however, is by nature heterogeneous and in some cases may be inactive (see Wampold et al., 2011). In primary care settings TAU could be quite active as it may be medication treatment or care by a primary care physician that is quite far from a waiting list condition, which in most cases is no treatment at all. In some cases evaluating CBT to the treatment provided in primary care settings provides the optimal test for efficacy when considering what treatment options ought to be provided. The following pages attempt to provide a clinician-friendly guide to the evidence base for CBT with older people.

CBT for Late Life Depression

CBT is the most extensively researched form of psychotherapy for late life depression (Laidlaw et al., 2003; Pinquart et al., 2006; Wilson et al., 2008). A lot of the data for the efficacy of CBT for late life depression were generated in the US in the 1980s and 1990s. However, many of these early intervention studies shared a number of significant flaws that may fail to meet criteria for modern clinical trials.

Many of these studies were conducted before the emergence of guidelines such as the CONSORT 2010 criteria (Consolidated Standards of Reporting Trials) or PRISMA, which are robust frameworks for the reporting of randomised controlled trial data and guidelines on the reporting of systematic reviews and meta-analyses. Some of the earlier studies recruit samples that are looking increasingly young in light of recent demographic changes (with entry into the studies from age 55 and mean ages of samples in the mid-60s). There are evident problems in the length of follow-up of evaluation, and many studies rely on the publication of 'completer' data rather than using intention to treat designs.

Recently, NHS Education for Scotland (NES) has developed a commissioning guide to the best evidence-based practice in terms of psychological interventions. The guide is known as *The Psychology Matrix*, and there is a section that reviews evidence for psychological interventions for depression and anxiety with older people, as well as dementia and long-term conditions psychological interventions with older people (NES, 2011).

In a recent meta-analysis, Hollon and Ponniah (2010) reviewed the outcomes of psychological therapies for mood disorders and found that CBT is efficacious

---

[2] LOCF (last observation carried forward) is a way of dealing with missing data in clinical trials (Gupta, 2011).

and specific in terms of treatment outcome. This is a positive result, as the review included CBT treatment trials conducted with older people. Cuijpers et al. (2009), in their recent meta-analysis, concluded that psychological therapy treatment outcomes are comparable for younger and older adults. What was interesting in the review by Cuijpers et al. (2009) is that many of the CBT trials with older people reported completer samples rather than using intention to treat designs (a much more conservative procedure as the data from people who do not complete treatment are incorporated into the data) and many of the earlier studies used quite young older people.

Two recent studies, conducted in the UK in primary care settings, merit further discussion as these data have corrected many of the methodological flaws evident in the earliest outcome studies in the US. The UK RCT studies (Laidlaw et al., 2008; Serfaty et al., 2009; 2011) both used an intention to treat design when reporting data and recruited much older participants than many of the earlier studies. In addition, the participants were recruited from UK NHS primary settings and were not recruited from university medical centres. Thus these studies represent a clinical population closest to those seen in routine clinical practice.

CBT for Late Life Depression: Individual Treatment Trial Data

In the first UK evaluation of individual CBT for late life depression in primary care, Laidlaw et al. (2008) randomly allocated participants to one of two treatment conditions: CBT alone or TAU. In the TAU condition, older participants received the range of treatments they would ordinarily receive in primary care, without external influence or pressure. Laidlaw et al. (2008) reported benefits in depression outcome for CBT alone and TAU, at the end of treatment and at six months follow-up. However, after taking account of baseline scores between the groups a significant difference in outcome emerged, with participants in the CBT treatment group recording significantly lower scores on the Beck Hopelessness Scale (which measures optimism and pessimism) at six months after the end of treatment, compared with participants in the TAU group. Moreover, significant differences favouring CBT also emerged on evaluation of the number of participants who remained depressed according to their Research Diagnostic Categorisation status (a way of systematically agreeing symptom-level measures of depression) at the end of treatment and at three months follow-up. Thus, although the study was small and the levels of depression mild, the findings suggest that CBT by itself (participants who received this treatment also did not receive medication) is an effective treatment for late life depression. This study remains one of the very few to compare the efficacy of psychological treatment with treatment usually offered in primary care, and one of the very few that has systematically measured the effectiveness of CBT as a treatment in a non-medicated treatment group.

Serfaty et al. (2009; 2011) provide further compelling evidence for the efficacy of CBT for late life depression in primary care populations. This study compared CBT plus TAU, a talking control condition plus TAU, and TAU alone. CBT participants on average achieved better treatment outcomes compared to the talking control condition and TAU, with 33 per cent of those receiving CBT recording a 50 per cent or greater reduction in BDI scores, compared to 23 per cent and 21 per cent, respectively, for those receiving TAU and the talking control treatment. Importantly, Serfaty et al. (2009) conclude their results discredit the myth that depressed older people are lonely and simply need a listening ear, as those in the talking control group did less well than those in the CBT treatment group. For readers interested in more detail about the talking control condition, Serfaty et al. (2011) provide a very interesting description.

There have been a number of systematic reviews and meta-analyses conducted since 2000 and the data for late life depression are summarised in Table 3.1. This table focuses on systematic reviews and meta-analyses rather than individual studies, as these tend to show more trends in outcome than may be seen in individual treatment studies. The data suggest that CBT consistently reports strong treatment outcomes in comparison to other forms of psychological therapy.

Some reviews report a statistical advantage for CBT compared to other forms of psychological intervention and with pharmacotherapy (Pinquart et al., 2006; 2007; Pinquart & Sorensen, 2001). There is evidence that CBT with older people is as efficacious as with adults of working age, although there are differences in the methodological quality of clinical trials with older people and in the main participants in late life clinical trials for depression tend to be relatively young and healthy, as is usual in clinical trial data from the US (Cuijpers et al., 2009; Gould et al., 2012a).

Overall, data from individual clinical trials (especially the more recent UK clinical data), systematic reviews and meta-analyses suggest CBT is the most efficacious psychological treatment approach for late life depression. A number of conclusions about the evidence base for CBT for late life depression are warranted:

- Efficacy of CBT in late life depression is stronger than for other forms of therapy, but there remains insufficient studies of optimal quality to definitively conclude that CBT is superior to other forms of psychological therapy in older people (Gould et al., 2012a; Wilson et al., 2008).
- Individual CBT treatment appears to be superior to group CBT interventions (Krishna et al., 2011; Pinquart et al., 2007).
- CBT appears comparable in efficacy to medication, in terms of both treatment outcome and drop-out, but the amount of data is very small as this comparison has rarely been undertaken with older people with depression (Pinquart et al., 2006).
- There are limited data examining the effect of combination treatments (i.e. CBT plus medication versus medication or CBT alone) in late life depression, and this is an area that needs further focus (Pinquart et al., 2007; Wilson et al., 2008).
- CBT is as efficacious with older adults as with younger adults, but the literature on psychotherapy outcome with the oldest-old (aged 75 years and above) is insufficient as many of the earlier outcome studies tended to recruit very 'young-old' participants, and with the change in demographics these data may no longer be appropriate (Cuijpers et al., 2009).
- Many of the earlier psychotherapy and CBT outcome studies tended to report data on completer samples rather than use intention to treat (ITT) designs, and hence results may be less conservative than would be optimal. Recent CBT outcome studies have reported efficacious outcomes when using ITT designs (Laidlaw et al., 2008: Serfaty et al., 2011).

TABLE 3.1 *Summary of evidence from systematic reviews of CBT for late life depression, 2000 onwards*

Authors	Level of analysis	Results	Conclusions
Laidlaw, 2001.	Focused review of 8 studies of CBT for late life depression (review of 5 meta-analyses in addition to outcome studies).	When using the BDI as the outcome measure, CBT showed the largest treatment gains in comparison to other psychological therapies. Many methodological flaws evident in earlier outcome studies.	CBT is an efficacious treatment for late life depression. Evidence supportive of this comes from outcome studies and from meta-analyses and systematic reviews.
Pinquart & Sorensen, 2001.	122 psychosocial intervention studies.	CBT and psychodynamic psychotherapy effective on self-rated and clinician-rated measures of depression. Individual therapy more effective than group.	The review considers a number of moderator variables that influence outcome, and notes that for CRD, longer duration of psychotherapy was more effective. For CRD there were larger improvements overall. Therapists with specialist training in older adults produced more effective outcomes.
Scogin et al., 2005.	20 studies selected comparing 6 evidence-based treatments identified as beneficial. Combination studies and maintenance treatments excluded from review.	The following treatments met criteria for evidence-based treatments: CBT, behaviour therapy, cognitive bibliotherapy, problem-solving therapy, brief psychodynamic therapy, and reminiscence therapy.	The most notable omission in this review is IPT. Many of the interventions need additional support as the numbers of studies are still relatively small, and most report data on 'young' older people (age 60–75 years). There is also limited evidence when looking at the combination of psychotherapy and pharmacotherapy.
Cuijpers, 2006.	25 studies, with 17 comparing psychotherapy with control condition.	Psychological therapies effective with older people. Broad inclusive approach to psychosocial interventions with moderate to large effect size (0.72) generated overall. No clear differences between different types of psychological therapies emerge.	The quality of studies included in the review was variable. Definitive conclusions for comparisons between medication and psychotherapy were not possible due to insufficient studies, but no overall differences in outcome were identified. There was some indication that combination of medication and psychological therapy was more effective than either alone, but the numbers of studies are small.

(Continued)

TABLE 3.1 *(Continued)*

Authors	Level of analysis	Results	Conclusions
Pinquart et al., 2006.	89 Studies (62 pharmacological; 32 psychological; 5 combination treatments). Major depressive disorder in 37 studies; 52 studies with mixed diagnoses.	For clinician-rated depression, 66 per cent of patients receiving pharmacotherapy and 72 per cent receiving psychotherapy showed above average improvement in outcome. For self-rated depression, 65 per cent of patients receiving pharmacotherapy and 69 per cent receiving psychotherapy showed above average improvement in outcome.	CBT more effective for depression in comparison to other medications and psychotherapies. Indications suggest that minor depression or dysthymia responds better to psychotherapy than pharmacotherapy. Few studies (5) compared treatments with a control condition. There is a paucity of studies conducted with the oldest-old (aged 75 years and above).
Pinquart et al., 2007	57 studies published between 1974 and 2006. 18/57 reported on major depressive disorder only, 37 mixed minor/major and dysthymia. Broad range of psychosocial interventions.	Pre-post-improvement on average was moderate for self-rated studies in participants with major depression and large in heterogeneous clinical symptoms. For clinician-rated depression effect sizes for treatment were large regardless of diagnostic status. There were no significant differences in attrition either for treatment approach or whether participants met diagnostic criteria for major depression.	In this review, IPT is included and reports a small effect size which is a great surprise; however, the number of studies evaluated in this review for this condition is very small and therefore caution is advised assessing this outcome. CBT and reminiscence studies record large effect sizes for outcome while other psychotherapeutic modalities (such as PP, psychoeducation, supportive approaches, etc.) report moderate effect sizes. Pinquart et al. (2007: 653) conclude that 'CBT and reminiscence, are efficacious in reducing depressive symptoms in older adults. Given that patients with physical or cognitive comorbidity are less likely to benefit from available psychotherapies, these patients warrant special attention in future research. . . . Our results indicate that the effectiveness of psychotherapy does not reduce with increasing age. Thus, general practitioners should pay more attention to the depressive symptoms of older adults and the possibility of treating them with psychotherapy.'

Authors	Level of analysis	Results	Conclusions
Wilson et al., 2008.	Cochrane Review with 82 randomised controlled trials of psychotherapy for late-life depression reviewed; 9 studies included in analyses. Overall, 12 studies included in the review (3 additional papers examined bibliotherapy). CBT was main treatment reviewed.	7 CBT studies and 2 psychodynamic psychotherapy studies were included in the review and analysis. 5 studies compared CBT with a waiting control condition. CBT was significantly more effective than waiting list controls with superior outcome for dropout of CBT compared to waiting list controls. Compared to active treatment controls CBT was superior in outcome. There was a mix of group and individualised interventions.	Overall, narrowness of review limits definitive conclusions as very few studies met criteria for inclusion. Although there is a paucity of good quality randomised controlled trials, CBT is an effective treatment with older people in comparison to active treatment controls and waiting list controls.
Cuijpers et al., 2009.	112 studies compared psychotherapy outcome between older adults and adults of working age. 20 studies involving older adult participants included in analyses.	The effect sizes of both groups did not differ significantly from each other (older adults: d = 0.74; younger adults: d = 0.67). Older adult and adult outcome studies report comparable effect sizes of 0.62, thus about 73 per cent of psychotherapy participants improved. The older adult studies were more heavily weighted towards completer analysis rather than ITT. In regression analyses there was no effect for age of participants thus outcome in psychotherapy studies between younger and older people are comparable.	There is no significant difference between psychotherapy outcome for adult versus older adult in the research literature. There are gaps in knowledge in terms of outcome of psychotherapy with older adults including severe depression and depression in the oldest-old. 'Although more research is needed on representative clinical samples, in older old adults, and in more severe forms of depression, our study shows that currently there is no reason not to apply psychotherapy for depression in old age' (Cuijpers et al., 2009: 23).

(Continued)

TABLE 3.1 (Continued)

Authors	Level of analysis	Results	Conclusions
Krishna et al., 2011.	Examined data for group-based psychotherapy interventions for late life depression. Of 360 papers screened, 296 were rejected, 64 were examined in detail and 6 were included in review. All 6 studies were CBT based	CBT effective with overall significant mean difference at p < 0.001. CBT was more efficacious than waiting-list conditions but not in comparison to active treatment control conditions. Gains in CBT were maintained at follow-up, although length of this was difficult to determine across studies included in review. Attrition between intervention and control groups non-significant.	Narrowness of review limits conclusions about group-based CBT efficacy as very few studies met criteria for inclusion. The quality of studies was not optimal as most of the effect size can be attributed to 3 of the 6 studies included in review. A number of the studies included young older adults in their trials.
Samad et al., 2011	Of 633 studies identified, 58 were examined for efficacy of behaviour therapy for depression in older people, but only 4 studies met inclusion criteria and all were published before 2000, with three published in the 1980s.	Results suggest BT = CBT & PP > W/L. There was a lot of heterogeneity in the 4 studies and hence the medium effect size of self-ratings (GDS, BDI) for BT vs W/L was not significant. When considering clinician-ratings there were significant differences between BT and W/L. There were no differences in treatment efficacy between BT and CBT with a slight non-significant advantage to CBT. Attrition rates varied in the 4 studies from 16 to 53 per cent.	A rather narrow review focusing on a small pool limits usefulness of conclusions. The data suggest the superiority of behaviour therapy over waiting lists but not compared to other active treatment conditions. 'The main findings from this review show that behavioural therapy for older people is significantly more effective than waiting list control when measured by clinician-rated depression using the HRDS, but not significantly different when measured by patient self-report . . . We also found that behavioural therapy is not significantly different in effectiveness compared with cognitive therapy or brief psycho-dynamic therapy whether using self-reported measures or clinician-rated assessment' (Samad et al., 2011: 1218).

Authors	Level of analysis	Results	Conclusions
Gould et al., 2012a.	485 studies of CBT with older people were examined and 23 were included in review. Most studies in this review used non-active controls (e.g. waiting list or treatment as usual[1]).	At the end of treatment CBT produced significant moderate pooled effect sizes (0.57) when compared to non-active treatment conditions, but there were no differences comparing CBT to other treatment conditions. At 6 months follow-up the same result was obtained with significant moderate pooled effect sizes (0.50) for CBT when compared to non-active treatment conditions.	This review incorporates contemporary recent RCTs not included by other reviews. However, this review seems somewhat naïve regarding the clinical realities in conducting trials. The authors correctly identify a number of flaws in the quality of the data most evidently from earlier studies. 'Overall, participants who received CBT had significantly greater odds of remitting or having clinically significant improvement than nonactive controls . . . Participants who received CBT did not have significantly greater odds of remitting than those who received other treatment' (Gould et al., 2012a: 1820).

[1] Treatment as usual (TAU) is considered non-active when in some cases this can be an active management in primary care and in some cases may indicate treatment using medication according to standard treatment protocols.

Notes: BT = behaviour therapy, CRD = clinician-rated depression, IPT = interpersonal psychotherapy, PP = psychodynamic psychotherapy, RCT = randomised controlled trials, W/L = waiting list

Summary: CBT for Late Life Depression

Treatment data for CBT with older people are very positive and serve to emphasise what most clinical geropsychologists know already: older people are by and large good candidates for CBT. In many respects we should not be surprised that CBT works well with older people, as older people tend to value the core principles of this treatment approach because it is skills enhancing, present oriented, problem focused and straightforward to use, as well as effective.

The overall conclusion about CBT with older people is that there is good evidence that it is effective for a range of common mental health problems, but many more studies need to be conducted in order to reach a more definitive conclusion. Conditions that are associated with age such as dementia, stroke and Parkinson's disease are being recognised as having significant psychological consequences for the individual and their caregivers. The evidence base for psychotherapies in these conditions reflects an emerging literature that is rich with promise (see Chapter 10).

Learning Log: Reflection and Review
What have you gained from reading this chapter?

- What are your thoughts about the prevalence and incidence of depression in later life? Are you surprised by these data? What impact could this information have on your practice? Make some notes on how you could use this information within your sessions with older people.
- Would you consider a small audit of referrals to your service, both in terms of presenting problems and in terms of source of referral? Can you or some of your colleagues look at treatment outcomes naturalistically? What outcome do you achieve, and how does this compare with the evidence base presented in the tables in this chapter?
- Do you have influence on the assessment measures and procedures used in your service? Can you review the use of measures to ensure that older adult-specific measures are being used where appropriate?

Further Reading

The following sources provide more in-depth coverage of topics raised in this chapter.

Cuijpers, P., van Straten, A., Smit, F., & Andersson, G. (2009). Is psychotherapy for depression equally effective in younger and in older adults? A meta-regression analysis. *International Psychogeriatrics, 21*, 16–24.

Lyness, J. (2007). Effects of psychotherapy and other behavioural interventions on clinically depressed older adults: a meta analysis. *Aging & Mental Health, 11*, 645–657.

Moher, D., Liberati, A., Tetzlaff, J., & Altman, D. G., The PRISMA Group (2009). Preferred reporting items for systematic reviews and meta-analyses: the PRISMA statement. *PLoS Med*, 6(7), e1000097. doi:10.1371/journal.pmed.1000097.

Scogin, F. & Shah, A. (Eds.). (2012). *Making evidence-based psychological treatments work with older adults*. Washington, DC: APA.

Four
CBT for Late Life Anxiety

Learning Objectives
By the end of this chapter you will:

- Learn about the prevalence of anxiety disorders in later life
- Become knowledgeable about measurement issues in late life anxiety
- Be able to select the most appropriate assessment measure for late life anxiety disorders in terms of diagnostic value, symptom severity, and utility as a measure of change
- Understand the efficacy data for CBT for anxiety disorders in later life

Anxiety in Later Life

Recent evidence suggests that anxiety disorders are very common in later life (Bryant et al., 2008) and may be more common than late life depression (Wolitzky-Taylor et al., 2010). Depression and anxiety often overlap in older people, but anxiety tends to be neglected and undertreated in primary care (Vink et al., 2008). When anxiety (either experienced as symptoms or disorder) is comorbid with a mood disorder, older people are more likely to come into contact with mental health services and more likely to be seen by mental health specialists, indicating severity and complexity of presentation (Scott et al., 2010). A mixed presentation of anxiety comorbid with depression may result in poorer treatment prognosis (Diefenbach & Goethe, 2006). Generalised anxiety disorder (GAD) frequently coexists with depression, and may be difficult to differentiate from depression. Whereas depression may have a recurrent course, GAD may present as a single chronic episode lasting years or even decades (Lenze et al., 2005).

Anxiety in older people may have long-term consequences in terms of physical and emotional health, yet it tends to go 'under the radar' of mental health professionals and even older people themselves, so that they are less likely to seek help with anxiety disorders (Scott et al., 2010) or to be offered treatment. In general, anxiety has been neglected in terms of its prevalence and impact on the mental health and well-being of older people (Lenze et al., 2005; Wetherell et al., 2005).

There are some interesting things to understand about anxiety when working with older people. First among these is that anxiety may not necessarily be a new feature in the lives of the older people with anxiety disorders that you meet in clinical practice (Lenze et al., 2005), although there is a lack of consensus on this and some researchers contend that late onset anxiety is not uncommon (Wetherell et al., 2005).

When older people experiencing panic symptoms are also diagnosed with physical illnesses this may complicate the picture. Therefore, when anxious older people with physical illnesses express concerns about their health this may be responded to by health professionals in a way that inadvertently reinforces responses such as maladaptive health-seeking behaviours in older people.

Case Example

Rowena[1] is a 78-year-old widow who lives on her own following the sudden death of her husband two years previously after a heart attack. As Rowena has smoked all her life (her husband was a smoker too) she has developed Chronic Obstructive Pulmonary Disease (COPD). In the evenings she has started to experience panic attacks and she phones the NHS 24 Helpline in a state of fear and alarm.

> Panic attacks are anxiety symptoms that come on suddenly 'out of the blue' and are usually highly distressing to the person experiencing them. The symptoms of a panic attack[2] include:
>
> Palpitations
> Sweating (not due to the heat)
> Chest pains
> Shortness of breath
> Nausea
> Stomach churning
> Dizziness
> Feeling faint
> A feeling of dread
> Shaking

When the phone operator hears Rowena describe her anxiety symptoms such as heart racing, chest pains, dizziness and feeling faint, she is regularly sent to accident and emergency (A&E) for assessment. Repeatedly, Rowena is taken by ambulance to A&E. This raises Rowena's sense of alarm and understandably makes her fear that something serious must be wrong with her heart. At the A&E department, Rowena's experience of waiting for tests and having an ECG assessment again convinces her that she is very

---

[1] Not her real name.

[2] Symptoms from NHS website: www.nhs.uk/Conditions/Panic-disorder/Pages/Symptoms.aspx

vulnerable and contributes to a set of developing safety behaviours where she will contact the NHS 24 Helpline if she is feeling unwell, or in anticipation of developing difficulties. As Rowena is convinced of her vulnerability, her conviction is strong that she will die unless she does something. In this scenario her behaviour is understandable. Her elevated anxiety level has an unfortunate impact on her breathing rate, and because of her COPD[3] her fears that she is in imminent danger are made more acute by breathing difficulties, so a vicious cycle is created and maintained.

> Helping older people to manage anxiety symptoms may be complicated by physical comorbidity. COPD is a good example. The physical symptoms can be disabling (chronic cough, excess sputum, breathlessness) and can be anxiogenic (increase anxiety and panic symptoms) (Baraniak & Sheffield, 2011).
>
> The symptoms of COPD are irreversible and chronic. Cognitions in COPD may not be helpful and may contribute to fear, worsening breathlessness in an ever-deteriorating fear cycle.
>
> CBT can be challenging to apply here. Remember in CBT the concept is that it is the individual's appraisal of their experience rather than the experience itself that is important in determining how an individual copes. This is very useful when working with people with COPD.

In part, Rowena's actions and responses are reinforced by the response of healthcare professionals. She has stopped going out for fear of exerting herself and causing herself more danger. During the day Rowena sits by the large picture window in her home and watches people passing by – she is reassured that there are people she could call to if the need arose. When she experiences panic attack symptoms during the day she will stand by her open front door and 'get more oxygen', and by these safety behaviours she is able to restrain herself from calling for help. What is notable about the times that Rowena calls for help is that these always occur in the evenings when she feels more alone.

Rowena had a strong independent streak and her reliance on others was a source of injury to her pride. CBT was useful to Rowena as it empowers people to effect change on their own terms. As it became clear that Rowena felt more vulnerable at night in response to the exact same set of symptoms, but would respond in different ways depending on the time of day, this allowed us to examine what motivated her behaviour. When we sat down and carefully worked out the strength of her belief that she was about to have a heart attack (using dysfunctional thought records), it became evident that despite her belief being 100 per cent at the time the fear never materialised as she was still alive despite her concerns. I would start our sessions by reviewing her previous week, and I would ask: 'So, Rowena, how many times have

---

[3] Evidence for CBT as an effective treatment for anxiety and depression in COPD is starting to emerge, with Hynninen et al. (2010), Kunik et al. (2001) and Kunik et al. (2008) all reporting potentially effective results.

you died this week?' This may seem rather stark, and may even seem unfeeling, but as it was said with a hint of humour and a large dose of empathy for the distress and fear experienced by Rowena, it got to the heart of the matter for her, as she understood her fears had become mixed with past experience and were acting to scare her into actions she knew were not necessary.

Rowena is worried that she may suddenly die like her husband and there will be no one there to help her. The therapist was careful to get Rowena to describe her most recent experiences of panic attacks in explicit and highly specific detail. At the peak of her panic, Rowena is 100 per cent certain that she will die. This is extremely frightening and her experience of her husband's sudden death reinforces her sense of vulnerability. Once Rowena and I shared this new understanding (feelings aren't facts, even things we believe in 100 per cent don't come true) we were able to modify Rowena's fear behaviours with a reduction in the frequency of attendance at A&E and a reduction in calls to the NHS 24 Helpline in the evenings.

This case example illustrates a number of key points about applying CBT with older people:

1. Anxiety or depression treatment may be complicated by a pre-existing physical comorbidity that may also complicate treatment, as the symptoms of the physical condition and their psychological consequences can become conflated.
2. When working with older people, you may also find that external factors, and the understandings and responses of other healthcare professionals, can in certain respects complicate diagnosis, assessment and treatment.
3. The extent of possible change may not be apparent until you start to explore this on an individual basis using behavioural experiments.
4. In some cases physical conditions are irreversible and may be deteriorating, therefore aims for therapy may become more fluid in response.
5. There is an important emphasis on keeping in mind a working hypothesis as to the psychological context, therefore frequently reviewed case-conceptualisations are helpful.
6. There is a temptation to treat cases like Rowena's with a more complex intervention when the reality is that what is required is basic CBT done to a high standard (i.e. stick to behaviour experiments and cognitive restructuring).

Assessment Tools with Older People: Measuring Anxiety in Later Life

When attempting to measure anxiety symptoms and levels of distress in older people, clinicians need to take account of the complication of assessing anxiety symptoms when there may be comorbid physical factors masking the true level of anxiety (see Dennis et al., 2007).

The Royal College of Psychiatrists' Faculty of the Psychiatry of Old Age (RCP, 2012) free assessment guideline for individual patient outcome measurement covers assessment tools in late life anxiety. For the assessment of anxiety in older people, the RCP (2012) recommend the HADS and the GAD-7. The HADS has been reviewed under the section on depression measures and there may be some concern as to its utility in assessing both depression and anxiety (Norton et al., 2013).

While evidence suggests that standard anxiety measures such as the Beck Anxiety Inventory (BAI), the Penn State Worry Questionnaire (PSWQ) and the GAD-7 are reliable and valid in assessing anxiety in older people (see Segal et al., 2010; Crittendon & Hopko, 2006), there are specifically developed self-report measures of anxiety disorder in older people – such as the Geriatric Anxiety Inventory (GAI) (Pachana et al., 2007) and the Geriatric Anxiety Scale (GAS) (Segal et al., 2010) – that hold particular promise and will be discussed in greater detail later in the chapter.

Many other assessments currently in use with older people were designed with adults of working age in mind but may not be entirely suitable. A very commonly used measure is the BAI (Beck et al., 1988).

Beck Anxiety Inventory (BAI; Beck et al., 1988)

The BAI (Beck et al., 1988) is a psychometrically robust 21-item self-report screening test considered to have good internal consistency and excellent discriminant validity, but has been criticised for the inclusion of somatic items that may inflate anxiety scoring when used with older clients (Edelstein et al., 2008; Yochim et al., 2011). There are concerns that the BAI may require different cut-offs for use with older people, but the exact quantification of these have not been adequately established (Dennis et al., 2007). Morin et al. (1999) found that the BAI has good overall psychometric properties, although there is a concern over the ability of the BAI to differentiate GAD from depression. This is a concern shared by Wetherall and Gatz (2005) when using the BAI with a sample of older people diagnosed with GAD. One needs to take account of the fact that there can be a lot of overlap between GAD and depression symptoms, and it would not be recommended to use a self-report assessment in place of clinical diagnosis and opinion.

Penn State Worry Questionnaire (PSWQ; Meyer et al., 1990)

The PSWQ is a 16-item self-report measure of worry rather than anxiety more generally. Originally developed by Borkovec et al. (Meyer et al., 1990) for use with adults of working age populations, it has nevertheless been used in a number of clinical trials of CBT with older people (see Wetherell et al., 2005). Stanley et al. (2001) suggest that the PSWQ reports good internal consistency, but questions remain regarding test-retest reliability. Crittendon and Hopko (2006) report on an abbreviated form of the PSWQ, comparing its more simplified format with students and community-dwelling older people. The format is simplified by removing negatively worded (reversed scored) anxiety items, thus potentially making this a more useful scale for people with Mild Cognitive Impairment (MCI). The PSQW-A ('A' for abbreviated) is a short version of the original PSQW. It is an 8-item self-report measure with a single underlying factor, suggesting it will be more focused as a measure of worry. Although the sample sizes are rather modest in this study, and the sample is not entirely representative of older people (mostly white, younger older people), the PSWQ-A reported strong internal consistency and excellent test–retest reliability, and may have some clinical utility when brevity of assessment is important.

Brief Measure of Generalised Anxiety Disorder (GAD-7; Spitzer et al., 2006)

The GAD-7 was developed by the same team who developed the PHQ-9 and, unsurprisingly, is also used for evaluating outcome (it is also a sensitive measure of change) as part of the IAPT initiative in the UK. It is also commonly used by GPs in primary care. Thus this measure will be very familiar to clinicians and may increasingly be used with older people. The GAD-7 is a simple 7-item scale originally derived from a larger 60-item scale, scored from 0 to 3 for each item so that a maximum score of 21 is obtained for the most severe experience of GAD. A score of 15 or more on this measure is considered a 'red flag', indicating a score that suggests treatment is warranted. A score of 10 indicates that further investigation is also warranted. Sorocco and Lauderdale (2011) suggest that the GAD-7 may be useful for use with older people, but provide no evidence to back this statement up. The GAD-7 has been validated for use with older people by Wild et al. (2013), who assessed the GAD-7 in a reasonably large community-dwelling sample of older people aged from 58 to 82 years of age. However, the number of people with diagnosable GAD was very small, suggesting caution in interpreting these data. Wild et al. (2013) recommend different cut-offs for the GAD-7 with older people, with scores of 5 and above optimal for sensitivity and specificity in detecting anxiety.

The Geriatric Anxiety Inventory (GAI; Pachana et al., 2007)

The GAI was developed as a specific measure of anxiety designed for use with older people in order to reduce the intrusion of somatic items in overall scaling. Many of the 20 items of the GAI appear to tap into worry-type domains, with fewer focusing on other domains in the range of anxiety disorders.

The GAI was originally developed with a sample of predominantly healthy community-dwelling older people and a smaller number of participants with GAD or worry. The GAI used a clinical sample in its development and in determination of cut-off scores. However, the clinical sample was exceptionally small, with only 24 per cent of this sample of mainly older women meeting current anxiety diagnoses.

The GAI has had a significant impact since its development, and it is rapidly becoming used as the measure of anxiety disorder in later life. However, as Yochim et al. (2011) point out, the GAI is probably more successful as a measure of worry, rather than being applicable to other anxiety disorders, as many of the items refer to this cluster of anxiety symptoms. In terms of its psychometric properties, it appears to evidence acceptable reliability and validity, with a single unitary factor structure for a 20-item scale. The GAI was modelled on the same structure and answer format as the GDS.

The GAI now has a short form (SF-GAI) (Byrne & Pachana, 2010). Based on 5 items of the original 20 in the GAI, the authors suggest that a cut-off of 3 is best for the detection of GAD. When looking at the items in the GAI-5 it seems the SF-GAI may function best as a measure of GAD symptoms. The development of a short form of the GAI is welcome, although clinicians may need to exercise caution in using this measure as it was developed entirely with a sample of women, the majority (90 per cent) of whom did not have any anxiety symptoms, as only eight (3 per cent) were diagnosed with GAD.

The Geriatric Anxiety Scale (GAS; Segal et al., 2010)

The GAS was developed in recognition of the need for an anxiety measure specific to older people that would avoid problems in adapting existing anxiety measures from other population groups. Segal and colleagues (Segal et al., 2010; Yochim et al., 2011) have produced a new, clinically useful scale that has been conceptually developed as a measure of late life anxiety. The GAS (Segal et al., 2010) is a 30-item scale (25 content items and 5 theme items not used for scoring) that has a 0–4 Likert scale response format. While not yet established in research, a Likert-report format, rather than a simple yes/no format, may make this method more suitable as a measure of change. Total scores can range from 0–75, with higher scores indicating problems with anxiety. The GAS is recommended, as it adds to the assessment 'toolbox' of clinicians by providing a measurement of anxiety that captures a more global and general anxiety profile, including cognitive, somatic and affective domains of anxiety. The ability to use an anxiety measure with older people that acknowledges and quantifies the somatic aspect of anxiety is very helpful. While no measure is ever perfect, and the GAS possesses significant strengths, there remain caveats to its use. The GAS is strongly and positively correlated with the GDS (thus a high score on the GAS would usually indicate a high score on the GDS), and it is developed with a modest sample size so psychometric aspects such as its factor structure remain to be fully explored. Yochim et al. (2011) compared the GAS with some other key tools such as the BAI and the GAI. The GAS correlated more strongly with the other anxiety measures (BAI, GAI) than either of these measures did with each other, reflecting perhaps the fact that the GAS provides a more comprehensive assessment of anxiety symptoms than either the GAI or BAI. The BAI tends to focus on somatic items of anxiety that may inflate scores and excludes affective components of anxiety, whereas the GAI tends to focus on worry affect in terms of anxiety (Yochim et al., 2011).

Key Messages about Late Life Anxiety

- Anxiety is under-recognised and undertreated. It may also be underappreciated for its impact in elevating risk of death and disability.
- Anxiety is probably more common than depression in older people but often presents comorbidly with depression.

- GAD and panic disorder with agoraphobia are the most common anxiety disorders.
- Prevalence is likely to be higher for anxiety symptoms than anxiety disorders in later life, and these are unlikely to spontaneously remit.
- There is a lack of consensus, but anxiety disorders are more likely to be early onset rather than late onset conditions. This has important implications for the application of psychological therapies.
- Assessment of anxiety disorders is quite complex, and while there are welcome additions of new measures specifically designed for use with older people no measure has yet established itself as a 'sufficient' general measure of anxiety, and therefore the GAD-7 (a more generic non-older adult tool) may be usefully augmented by the GAS or GAI depending upon the population worked with.

The most common anxiety disorder in later life is GAD, and as a result many of the outcome studies have evaluated treatment outcome for this disorder. There are a much smaller number of studies that have evaluated psychological therapies for panic disorder in later life, and even less have evaluated treatment for obsessive compulsive disorder (OCD) and post-traumatic stress disorder (PTSD). PTSD for World War II trauma has been evaluated and shown to be possibly effective, however, this cohort of older people are now less likely to present at clinics.

Highly specialised CBT for anxiety in people with executive dysfunction is a newly developed intervention that shows promise. In a pilot evaluation of CBT for late life anxiety, Mohlman and Gorman (2005) showed that outcome for CBT was poor in older adults with low levels of executive functioning abilities, but outcome improved for individuals classified as having low levels of executive functioning when their deficits in executive functioning were targeted and ability in this domain improved. Results from this small pilot study suggest CBT outcome may be enhanced if executive dysfunction is targeted for improvement via the use of attention training and enhanced self-monitoring rehabilitation skills classes (Mohlman & Gorman, 2005).

Data pertaining to CBT for late life anxiety disorder have been criticised because the studies have tended to be conducted with a generally young (aged 55 and over) older adult group of healthy and active volunteers with studies conducted in university settings (Hendriks et al., 2008). A recent RCT by Stanley et al. (2009) has answered many of these criticisms in a study conducted in primary care settings that shows a good outcome.

CBT, considered the gold-standard psychotherapy for anxiety disorders in adults of working age (Otte, 2011), appears to be less effective with older people because CBT (Gould et al., 2012b) for GAD is twice as effective with adults of working age compared to older people and attrition rates in GAD treatment trials are twice as high in older people (Gorenstein & Papp, 2007). There may not be a difference in the rates of treatment response for anxiety between older and younger adults however, because in some cases the evidence for CBT for GAD with working age adults might be somewhat overstated. For instance, a recent evaluation of CBT versus placebo for a range of anxiety disorders in working age adults by Hoffman and Smits (2008) note that GAD outcome for CBT is poorer than for other anxiety disorders (except panic disorder) when compared to a placebo.

Perhaps a more useful comparison is to examine the effectiveness of CBT for late life GAD with the data for CBT for GAD in working age adults. Aspinall (2013) examined the evidence for CBT used in the treatment of GAD in 39 studies reporting outcomes in adults of working age participants compared to outcomes achieved with older people. Aspinall (2013) reports no difference in effect sizes, with CBT involving older people being equally as efficacious as with adults of working age for GAD. Therefore, contrary to popular opinion, no significant difference appears to exist between the effectiveness of CBT for GAD based on age. Perhaps this intriguing result, based on over 1,500 participants in the pooled results, suggests that CBT for GAD could do better. Stated simply, GAD is a difficult condition to treat using brief CBT, as it has a longstanding history for the individual and requires a significant change in response to stressors

Lenze et al. (2005) examined the naturalistic course of GAD in older people, and reported that 46 per cent had a late onset of GAD (when aged 60 or over), but also that generalised anxiety rarely spontaneously remits. Thus, the mean duration of GAD was seventeen years, but 82 per cent experienced a continuous episode of GAD. Given the foregoing, it would appear that GAD is a condition that can challenge the quality of life for an individual and is likely to be challenging to treat effectively with a brief course of psychotherapy. The longevity associated with GAD suggests that this condition could become entrenched within individuals – this can be very challenging to treat with older people as a number of aspects of the cognitions and behaviours associated with this condition may have become inadvertently reinforced by significant others *and* healthcare professionals.

CBT Efficacy for Late Life Anxiety

The majority of studies evaluating CBT for anxiety disorders have been conducted in the US, and many have recruited participants from university-affiliated mental health centres and used recruitment via media announcements, and in some cases self-referral. The participants in clinical trials may therefore be very different from those found in routine clinical practice, and possibly different from anxiety treatment trials recruiting adults of working age. While some studies recruited participants with mixed anxiety disorders, most have focused on evaluating CBT for GAD. The quality of studies also varies, with some comparing CBT to waiting times, or to active conditions such as relaxation or supportive counselling. The mode of delivery of therapy also varies, with some studies using group approaches whereas others utilise individualised psychotherapy. This can contribute to a heterogeneous picture in terms of outcome and comparison across trials. Wetherell et al. (2005: 891) summarise the gaps in research outcome for psychological therapy for late life as follows:

Across the majority of clinical trials conducted to date, samples of patients are relatively homogeneous and often are not representative of older adults in general with regard to age, functional status, ethnicity, education or mental health … Relatively few data have addressed the value of treatment in more real-world settings, with patients who represent a broad range of demographic and clinical characteristics.

CBT for late life anxiety disorders report beneficial outcomes compared to waiting list controls (moderate effect sizes are the norm). However, results are less impressive when CBT is compared to active conditions (Gould et al., 2012b; NICE, 2012). In their review of CBT efficacy for late life anxiety, Ayers et al. (2007) make some interesting observations about earlier outcome studies that mainly use group CBT as a treatment for late life anxiety, with some aspects of treatment protocols limited because of this. Additionally Ayers et al. (2007) suggest that individual CBT may be a more optimal treatment approach because of the more idiosyncratic nature of fears. Hence treatment outcome may be limited because of methodology rather than anything to do with the age of the participants.

A further explanation of poorer treatment outcomes for CBT for anxiety disorders in later life can also be found in the complexity and continuity of anxiety problems among older people. Older people often experience poorer health than adults of working age, and this may complicate treatment outcomes for anxiety given that it can be difficult to separate the physical symptoms of illnesses from anxiety symptoms (Bryant et al., 2008; Wolitzky-Taylor et al., 2010).

When anxiety disorders are comorbid with depression, a poorer treatment outcome is likely, with a longer treatment response time and greater chronicity (Lenze et al., 2005). Mixed anxiety and depression in later life are more complex to treat and the efficacy of psychological therapies for this clinical presentation is not yet established.

Two randomised controlled trials conducted by Barrowclough et al. (2001) and Stanley et al. (2009) in the US, recruiting from primary care, have corrected some of the gaps in the outcome literature for CBT. Barrowclough et al. (2001) recruited somewhat older samples with some chronic physical comorbidity evident, although the mean age of participants still remains within the young-old category. This study compared CBT to active treatment control and reported an impressive superiority of CBT at end of treatment and follow-up. The study by Stanley et al. (2009) used ITT analyses as well as completer analyses and reported potentially impressive results, but again this study recruited younger, healthier and well-educated participants, the majority of whom appear to have self-referred into the trial, thus calling into question how generalisable this sample is with clients in primary care settings not affiliated with universities. Consequently, there remains a need for more robust treatment trials examining the efficacy of CBT as a treatment for late life anxiety in populations more representative of the client groups presenting in primary care settings. The evidence of psychological therapies for late life anxiety disorders is reviewed in Table 4.1.

NICE clinical updates for psychological treatment of anxiety disorders (NICE, 2012) take evidence for CBT for GAD in later life from two systematic reviews (Gould et al., 2012b; Goncalves & Byrne, 2012). These reviews are mixed, in that the former looks exclusively at psychotherapy and the latter looks at psychotherapy and pharmacotherapy. All reviews have some degree of subjectivity, despite the adoption of good

TABLE 4.1 *Empirical evidence from systematic reviews and meta-analyses of CBT for late life anxiety disorders*

Authors	Level of analyses	Results	Conclusions
Nordhus & Pellesen, 2003	First quantitative review of CBT for late life anxiety. 15 studies entered into review. Review is broad and inclusive. Studies classified as pre-post treatment with no control condition or as controlled trials with one other control condition. Most participants in clinical trials are physically robust.	7 out of 15 studies recruit participants with diagnosable anxiety disorder. Mean age not reported in 3 out of 15 studies, but overall mean age was 69.5 years. Overall, three-quarters of participants are female. Moderate mean effect size reported for all studies in review (0.55). Studies comparing psychological therapy to active control condition report small effect size (0.24), whereas when compared to no-treatment or wait-list moderate to large effect sizes (0.73) are reported.	CBT is an efficacious treatment for late life anxiety. Earlier research is sampled, hence there are a number of significant flaws in reported studies. Much heterogeneity is evident in clinical severity and in methodology comprising relevance to clinical settings with older people with physical and psychological comorbidity. Many studies report inadequate data on longer-term follow-up, so data on efficacy only applies to end of treatment outcome.
Ayers et al., 2007.	77 studies identified and 17 entered into review as they met inclusive evidence-based treatment (EBT) criteria. Studies were heterogeneous with respect to diagnostic status. Interventions were predominantly group-based. Participants' minimum age was 55. Participants had GAD or mixed anxiety disorder.	10 out of 17 studies evaluated CBT/CT and supported efficacy. 7 of the CBT cases with older people diagnosed with GAD reported a good outcome. 2 studies did not support efficacy for CBT. Relaxation was supported in 4/17 studies examining this option, although participants had subjective anxiety complaints rather than a diagnosable anxiety disorder. SP used as a comparison in three treatment trials. Some evidence for SP but not superior to CBT/CT.	Four EBTs (CBT, relaxation, SP and CT) meet criteria for efficacy as a treatment for late life anxiety. As with the earlier reviews, a number of studies recruit young older people (age 55+) and relatively healthy populations, thus the profile of participants in reviews may not translate directly to UK clinical populations. 'Many studies used group rather than individual treatment. Given the diversity of anxiety-related thoughts and the complexity of the cognitive restructuring procedure, it is perhaps not surprising that group relaxation training appears to be more effective than group cognitive therapy. Individual cognitive therapy may be more efficacious because it allows a more idiographic approach to assessment and treatment' (Ayers et al., 2007: 13).

Authors	Level of analyses	Results	Conclusions
Hendriks et al., 2008.	56 studies originally identified but only 7 studies (overall pooled 'n' = 398) met inclusion criteria. Included studies must utilise Randomised Controlled Trial methodology, and meet DSM-IV diagnostic criteria for an anxiety disorder. They primarily examined CBT outcome and participants aged 60 years and over.	Robust review of CBT vs active/passive control conditions. 4 CBT studies overall are efficacious when compared with wait list controls. SMD/ES of 0.44 favouring CBT. 5 CBT studies are overall efficacious compared with active controls. Effect size of 0.51 favouring CBT. CBT is not more effective in comparison to active control conditions in reducing worrying but there was a trend favouring CBT. Much of the efficacy generated by 2 studies. Most of the data are based on completer samples and there are no analyses possible based on follow-up data.	Data is analysed using Cochrane Review software. Perhaps, as a result, this rather narrow meta-analysis provides limited conclusions on a small data set. The authors conclude: 'The present meta-analysis shows the efficacy of CBT in the treatment of anxiety disorders (as based on DSM-IV criteria) occurring later in life. Not only was its efficacy demonstrated in various samples of over-60s when compared with a wait-list condition, it was also shown relative to an active control condition' (Hendriks et al., 2008: 407).
Thorp et al., 2009.	19 studies identified from 83 journal articles. Inclusion criteria shares the same flaws as earlier reviews in order to accommodate studies for review. Mixed anxiety disorders (8 studies focus on GAD) but also mixed diagnosis; e.g. structured diagnosis to subjective anxiety complaints. 4 studies had no control comparison.	8 out of 19 studies focused on GAD, 5 were mixed, 1 was Parkinson's disease and 5 were subjective anxiety complaints. Three Treatment options examined: CBT, wait list and CBT with RT. All active treatments were more efficacious than wait list or no treatment, but CBT not more effective than active conditions. Efficacy of relaxation training was not augmented by use of CBT in reduction of anxiety.	CBT was effective in treating late life anxiety. CBT with RT was more efficacious than active control conditions but not more efficacious on its own. Data difficult to interpret as studies included in review were heterogeneous in terms of diagnostic status and treatment modality. The authors conclude: 'The results must be interpreted with caution because of methodological limitations of analyses based on a small number of studies, differences in sample selection, and diverse control conditions (when controls were used). We suggest that in order to strengthen this nascent literature, psychotherapy studies of late-life anxiety should include active comparison conditions whenever possible' (Thorp et al., 2009: 112).

(Continued)

TABLE 4.1 *(Continued)*

Authors	Level of analyses	Results	Conclusions
Goncalves & Byrne, 2012.	Systematic review of pharmacotherapy and psychotherapy for GAD. 98 studies originally identified reduced to 30 for closer review and 20 studies entered into review. GAD was primary diagnosis and intervention was psychotherapy or pharmacotherapy. Drug trials tended to be larger than psychotherapy trials but had shorter treatment times. Drug treatments were very heterogeneous. No studies were identified that combined psychotherapy with pharmacotherapy for GAD in later life.	Pharmacotherapy trials report effect sizes of 0.32 (moderate). Psychotherapy trials report effect sizes of 0.33 (moderate). Consistent with other reviews, psychotherapy outcomes better in comparison to non-active control/no-treatment conditions. Pre-post improvement on average was moderate for self-rated studies in participants with GAD and for clinician-rated anxiety outcome in both psychotherapy and pharmacotherapy studies. There were no significant differences in attrition between physical and psychological treatments.	Robust review affording comparison of differential effectiveness of psychotherapy and pharmacotherapy. Response definition was heterogeneous as were attrition rates. Pharmacotherapy outcomes were also heterogeneous. The authors conclude: 'Psychotherapy was a more effective intervention for late-life GAD than wait list, usual care or minimal contact conditions, but the effect was lost when other active conditions were employed as comparators … caution is required when interpreting these results, as there were relatively few studies and they were likely to have been underpowered to detect superiority of one effective psychological treatment over another' (Goncalves & Byrne, 2012: 9).
Gould et al., 2012b.	356 CBT studies identified and 12 included in review. 9 out of 12 were conducted in North America. GAD was most common condition in 7 out of 12 studies.	CBT reported moderate effect sizes (0.66) compared to wait list controls. CBT reported small effect sizes (0.20) compared to active control conditions.	This review suggests that CBT is efficacious for late life anxiety disorders. The review is limited in conclusions because of small numbers. Nonetheless, there is a recognition of the need for more robust treatment trials in the area that permit examination of complexity and chronicity evident in later life.

Authors	Level of analyses	Results	Conclusions
	Half of the studies (6) used an active control condition. 11 out of 12 reported follow-up at 6 months. Methodological quality was somewhat poor. There was a mix of group and individualised interventions.	At 6 months follow-up CBT reported small to moderate effect sizes (0.29) compared to active control conditions. It was not possible to compare CBT to wait list controls at 6 months follow-up. In the small number of studies with sufficient data, at 12 months follow-up CBT reported small effect sizes (0.21) compared to active control conditions.	The authors conclude: 'Meta-analyses showed that, at 0-month follow-up, CBT was significantly and modestly more effective at reducing anxiety symptoms than treatment as usual or being on a wait list, although the between-group difference in effect size with active control was not statistically significant, and the effect size was small. At 6- but not 3- or 12-month follow-up, CBT was significantly more effective at reducing anxiety symptoms than an active control, but the effect size was small' (Gould et al., 2012b: 226).

Notes: Tx = treatment, CT = cognitive therapy, RT = relaxation training, SP = supportive psychotherapy.

ES = effect size, which quantifies the strength of differences between two groups on a common scale. According to Cohen (1992) an ES of 0.2 is small, 0.4 is moderate and 0.8 is large. It is very commonly used in examining the magnitude of difference between treatments in systematic reviews and meta-analyses.

SMD = standardised mean difference, a way of comparing different measures on a comparable scale or metric: i.e., if studies use different measures of anxiety comparing their differences is only possible if all means are converted to the same common scale or metric. SMD is used as an effect size and is also known as Cohen's *d* (Faraone, 2008).

standards from Cochrane and PRISMA, and have to contend with heterogeneity of trials, hence NICE (2012) concludes that more research is needed into psychotherapy for late life anxiety disorders but as yet makes no specific recommendations for older people other than recommending that they are offered the same treatment options as adults of working age.

The evidence base for late life anxiety in CBT appears problematic as treatment is not yet fulfilling its potential, but understanding the data is complex as there are many additional factors to consider when assessing outcomes contextually. In summary, the following statements are probably warranted:

- CBT appears less effective with older people compared to use with adults of working age (AWA) (Hunot et al., 2010). However, many studies use group rather than individual treatment (Ayers et al., 2007; Gorenstein & Papp, 2007; Wetherell et al., 2005).
- Most RCTs are small, use younger, relatively healthy well-educated older adults conducted in university medical clinics and appear to report completer data (Hunot et al., 2010; Wetherell et al., 2005). There is a need to develop clinical trials with oldest-old participants and for a broader range of anxiety disorders (Hendriks et al., 2008).
- Most trials have focused on GAD, with much more limited evidence for simple phobias, OCD, PTSD and Parkinson's disease (Ayers et al., 2007; Hendriks et al., 2008; Wetherell et al., 2005; Wolitzky-Taylor et al., 2010).
- Case study reports rarely report schematic and age-appropriate conceptualisations. We simply don't have enough studies conducted with older people with anxiety disorders that are chronic and complex and more representative of patients in real-world settings (Laidlaw, 2013c).

Summary: CBT for Late Life Anxiety Disorders

There remains much to be done to ensure that older people receive efficacious treatments and experience access comparable to that enjoyed by adults of working age (Laidlaw, 2013b). In particular, many older people with anxiety disorders may not receive appropriate treatments (Hendriks et al., 2008). We can be confident that CBT is efficacious with older people, but many simply do not have ready access to psychological therapies. Thus, more access to efficacious treatments needs to be one of the priorities of any mental health service and a key priority for primary care providers.

Learning Log: Reflection and Review
What have you gained from reading this chapter?

- What has surprised you about the prevalence, incidence and presentation of anxiety disorders in later life? Make a list of questions you need to answer to enhance your ability to work with clients with anxiety disorders.
- Review a recent case where you worked with someone with anxiety. Did the outcome match your expectations? Are there learning objectives from this case you can address before you work with your next client?

- Reread the case example involving the client with COPD. Are there additional learning needs when working with clients with physical problems? Is there a risk assessment you may wish to review?
- Do you have influence on the assessment measures and procedures used in your service? Can you review the use of measures to ensure that older adult-specific measures are being used where appropriate?

Further Reading

The following sources provide more in-depth coverage of topics raised in this chapter.

Allgulander, C. (2012). Generalized anxiety disorder: a review of recent findings. *Journal of Experimental and Clinical Medicine*, *4*, 88–91.

Bryant, C., Jackson, H., & Ames, D. (2008). The prevalence of anxiety in older adults: methodological issues and a review of the literature. *Journal of Affective Disorders*, *109*, 233–250.

Gorenstein, E. E. & Papp, L. A. (2007). Cognitive behavior therapy for anxiety in the elderly. *Current Psychiatry Reports*, *9*, 20–25.

Moher, D., Liberati, A., Tetzlaff, J., & Altman, D. G., The PRISMA Group (2009). Preferred reporting items for systematic reviews and meta-analyses: the PRISMA statement. *PLoS Med*, *6*(7), e1000097. doi:10.1371/journal.pmed.1000097.

Scogin, F. & Shah, A. (Eds.). (2012). *Making evidence-based psychological treatments work with older adults*. Washington, DC: APA.

PART 2
The Application of CBT with Older People

Five

Structure and Content of CBT with Older People

Learning Objectives
By the end of this chapter you will:

- Have learned about the structure of CBT for use across sessions and within different phases of treatment
- Be knowledgeable about how to assess whether your practice is consistent and within therapeutic modality
- Understand the importance of specific aspects of CBT such as homework
- Understand how to end CBT sessions with older people and how to achieve this in a collaborative manner

Introduction: A Consistent, Structured Treatment

CBT is a uniquely structured format of psychological therapy. Each CBT session should share the same elements. These include agenda setting, review of previous homework tasks, focus on current problems/session targets involving both cognitive restructuring and behavioural experiments, and the ending of sessions after agreement of new homework tasks. Some therapists appear to pick and choose the aspects of CBT structure they will accommodate in their practice, such as the use of agenda setting or utilising homework tasks at the end of every session, but this is almost always a mistake as it dilutes the efficacy of this treatment, and can result in confusion and dissatisfaction on the part of the client if elements are sometimes introduced and then withdrawn.

Structure Within CBT

CBT has a recognisable structure that sets it apart from other therapies. The basic procedural elements of CBT with older people are as follows:

1. Use Agendas at the Beginning of Each Session

Agenda setting is where the therapist and patient agree a plan for therapy. It is explicit and concrete.

Specific agendas depend on several factors such as stage of therapy, problems, levels of severity of depression, risk factors, etc.

- The therapist helps the patient develop an agenda

Agreeing an agenda at the start of therapy is important in determining what is discussed in therapy and to ensure that a consistent focus is maintained upon the patient's main problems.

This can be especially useful for maintaining a working focus in sessions with older clients who may otherwise do a lot of story telling during sessions, or become quite tangential in their conversations. Many therapists fear being seen as disrespectful and allow the client to talk without interruption, often losing the focus entirely. However, by referring to the agenda and using some humour to avoid interruptions being perceived as rude, older people can be helped to stay on track with information in session (Laidlaw et al., 2003).

Some therapists worry that agenda setting is cold, clumsy and interrupts the flow of what the person will say at the start of the session. However, an agenda for the session can usually be discussed and agreed within *three minutes* at the start of the session. Setting aside time at the start of the session to agree targets and to ensure the most pressing of the client's problems are being discussed within the relatively brief session is an *important* and *respectful* way to approach clients. If the agenda has a number of points then ask client to help you *prioritise*. You can set aside agreed amounts of time in your session to work through each priority. Be sure to stick with this agreement or your client may feel dissatisfied that you were unable to talk about their priorities.

The following gives an example of how to agree an agenda, with a typical approach as follows;

- *Probe question* – enquiring how the client has managed/coped since previous session

  'How have you been since last time?' (If a crisis or problem has developed in the interim the therapist may ask the client if they wish to discuss this in today's session.)

- *Bridging question* – bridge between sessions (what has the person thought about what was discussed last time?)

  'When you thought about our last meeting, did you have any specific concerns, or did anything occur to you that you might want to discuss further today?'

- *Review* and discussion of completed *homework* task

  'I wonder how you got on with the task we set for today? How did you get on with the homework task we agreed last time?'

Please note that clients frequently start talking about the homework, and you need to be careful to stop this initial summary of how they have coped with the homework merging into a start of the session prior to the agenda being set. It is important to stop the client by saying something such as:

  'Okay, that's great that you did the homework, but before we look at it further let's make a plan to make the best use of the time we have together today, and then we'll come back to the homework.'

- *Review* and agree the *main topic(s)/problem(s)* discussed *within the session*

  'What are the main things we ought to talk about today?' If the client cannot state any problems, the therapist can help the client reflect and review by asking 'when you were making your way here, or when you were sitting in the waiting area prior to our appointment, what things did you think we ought to look at today?'

- *Alternatively*, the therapist can ask:

  'If you think about the thing that is causing you most distress in your life what would that be, and can we talk about that today?'

Once the agenda has been agreed it is always important for the therapist to check with the person that the agenda covers the most important issues they are dealing with currently. For example:

  'If we talk about these issues (summarise topics) is there anything important we would miss out? Are we covering the most pressing and important problem areas your life right now?' Once that has been agreed and addressed it is important to return to discussing homework completion as the first part of the session. 'Okay, good, well lets talk about the homework, so you were saying ...'

Using Agendas with New Clients

As it is often important to start each new case as you mean to go on, it is recommended that you start your first session with an agenda and that you name this process for your client as their first introduction to CBT. For example, a typical start to a session might see the therapist ask the following:

  'Let me introduce myself, I am Dr ... , Your doctor has asked me to see you and I thought today we might want to talk about the problems you've been experiencing over the last few months or so, or even longer if you think that is important. I'd like to set some time aside before we finish to let you know about the type of therapy I use, it's called CBT, and after that we can decide together whether you'd like to continue working with me. Does that sound okay? ... Good, what I have just done is set our agenda for today. We need to make sure we always make the best use of the limited time we have together, so that's why it's important to always set an agenda at the start of our appointments. Okay, so what would you say are your main problems or difficulties.'

In the above interaction, the therapist has laid out the problem-focused nature of CBT straight away. The emphasis is also collaborative, as the therapist suggests that at the end of the session the therapist and patient can decide together whether to continue with therapy. This is empowering and suggests respect from the therapist to the patient. The predominantly ahistorical nature of CBT is hinted at when the therapist suggests that the time frame for discussion is relatively recent: 'over the last few months'. With patience and practice, agenda setting becomes second nature on the part of a CBT therapist.

2. Adopt a Psychoeducational Stance

In order for a client to become an equal partner in therapy, they often need education about the psychological approaches to understanding their difficulties. In time, the client becomes their own therapist (Beck, 2011).

3. Remember – Therapy is Time-Limited

All too often it is unclear to the client or even the therapist when the end of treatment has been reached, because there has been a failure *early on* to agree goals for treatment outcome. From session one onwards an agreement is made that as therapy progresses the outcomes will be reviewed on a regular basis. It is often helpful and reassuring to the person if you agree to review therapy progress after six sessions.

(3a) Socialising People to the Cognitive Model

At its most basic, socialising people to the cognitive model is really alerting clients (often for the first time) to the connections between thought and mood. Socialising clients should not become a long-winded lecture, but should be a clear and simple explanation making use of the client's own experiences if at all possible. An introduction to the 'hot cross bun' model linking thoughts, feelings, behaviours and physical state can be very helpful. For example;

'The approach I think may be helpful for you in dealing with x [either state explicitly a problem (behaviour), or list a set of problems identified collaboratively in session], is cognitive behaviour therapy, usually known as CBT. Have you heard of it at all? There has been a lot of research showing CBT to be helpful for people with the types of problems/symptoms you've described. The basic idea in CBT is that the way we think about something determines how we feel about it, and that can often impact on how we behave. Let me show you what I mean by using an example from something you brought into our session today.'

At this point the therapist can use an example from their client that links thoughts–feelings–behaviour, and it is helpful to work with the client to physically draw a diagram making these connections (see Figure 5.1, the hot cross bun model). It can be useful to set this out as a shared process:

'I'd be really interested in whether or not you think it is relevant to your difficulties and whether it makes sense to you. The way we think about things is important for making sense of how we feel about things that happen to us, and in understanding (and in some cases predicting) how we respond in certain situations. Let me show you what I mean.'

It is often very important to help your client identify the connection between their psychological and physical state. Using a sheet of paper you can enlist your client's help in completing the connections between each element of the model in Figure 5.1.

An example of a completed 'hot cross bun' is as follows: Jennifer is a 68-year-old retired widow who lives on her own and has reasonably good contact with her two adult children. She has recently taken on a 'rescue dog' from a charity, but she is finding it somewhat more challenging than she expected and feels unable to cope, especially as she has decided to have the dog 'rehoused'. She says that 'he's a lot of work and more boisterous than I bargained for. What a mess I make of my life. I make these decisions and I can't cope with them'. A way forward here is to use the hot cross bun model to educate your client about the impact of her negative statements – working with your client to make the connections, draw out the hot cross bun in Figure 5.2.

The important point here is to let the person see the reciprocal nature of connections between thoughts, feelings, behaviour and their physical state. It is important to point out to your client that they can change the way they think about things and

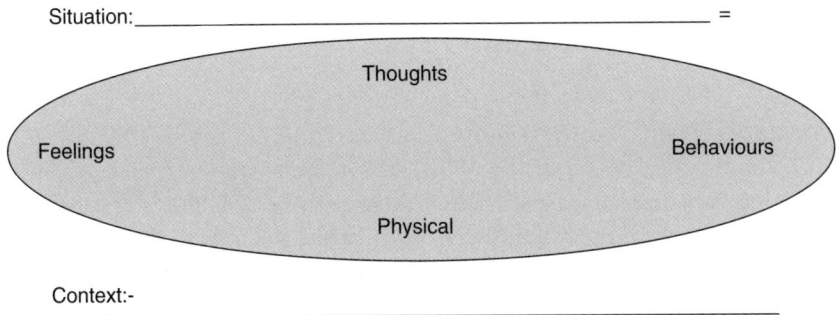

FIGURE 5.1 *The hot cross bun model for CBT, linking thoughts, feelings, behaviour and physical state*

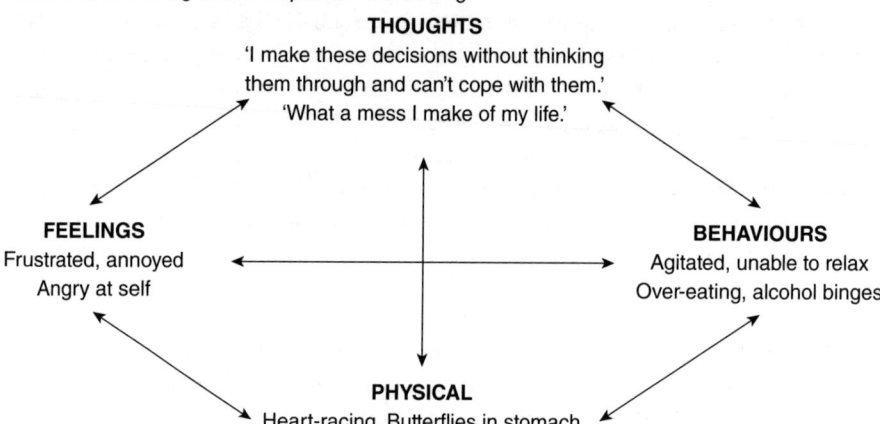

Situation: *Not being able to cope with rescue dog.*

THOUGHTS
'I make these decisions without thinking
them through and can't cope with them.'
'What a mess I make of my life.'

FEELINGS
Frustrated, annoyed
Angry at self

BEHAVIOURS
Agitated, unable to relax
Over-eating, alcohol binges

PHYSICAL
Heart-racing, Butterflies in stomach
Tightness in chest, insomnia

Context: *Habitual negative self-appraisal style: Often self-blaming and punitive.*
Unforgiving of self but very understanding towards others.

FIGURE 5.2   *The hot cross bun model as an aide to socialising people to CBT*

the way they behave. If these are connected to their feelings and to their physical state then these elements must change too.

The hot cross bun model can serve as an introductory working hypothesis of the underlying (covert) nature of the client's problems, and is very useful for getting an early indication of where challenges for client, therapist and dyad may lie. For Jennifer, there seems to be an issue about self-defeating behaviours demoralising her and undermining her sense of agency. As the therapist and client work together and discuss the connections they have made with relevance to an actual example from the client, the therapist may find it useful to summarise a way of understanding things from a CBT perspective:

> 'Our ways of thinking can become unhelpful to us. CBT involves understanding these unhelpful thinking patterns and the impact they have on our emotions and we learn new ways to manage situations better. In CBT we like to think that if we work together to understand and solve your problems in this way, you'll be better equipped in the future to manage any challenges that might come your way. How does that sound to you?'

4. Measurement is Important

Often clients have unrealistic expectations for change that may in the early stage of therapy interfere with the process of recovery. Often clients will monitor their progress but, as they are still depressed or anxious, the amount of progress made is usually viewed from a skewed baseline such that clients frequently fail to notice progress in treatment. It is therefore extremely important to build-in some monitoring or evaluation method from the first session onward (for appropriate measures see Chapters 3 and 4). The frequency of measurement may depend on a number of factors, but as a minimum it is recommended that baseline, mid-point and end of treatment measures are made so as to gauge progress during treatment. As CBT is an individualised treatment you may wish to augment the use of measurement with a more personalised measurement tool, such as a visual analogue of progress on a variable important to the client.

5. Use Socratic Questioning

The primary means of exploration within sessions is to use *Socratic questioning*. This is a specific format adopted for data gathering within the structure of CBT sessions. Socratic questioning does not involve the therapist following a 'roadmap', taking a client on a journey from their perspective about situations to the 'right' destination answer (i.e. from A to B). On the contrary, Socratic questioning involves a joint process of exploration and discovery between client and therapist, where the destination and elements of the journey are unknown at the outset, that is, from A to wherever (Laidlaw, 2008a). In this way the client can be encouraged to look afresh at their attributions for events and how helpful this is for them.

Socratic questioning in therapy uses explorative open-ended questions. It means that the therapist adopts an assumption-free approach to understanding their client. In order that clients are fully understood, therapists need to maintain a stance towards exploration in therapy rather than interpretation.

> Use Socratic questioning sensitively, as clients often assume that the therapist knows the 'correct' answer but is withholding until they have 'guessed' it (Bishop & Fish, 1999).

It is important to focus in on the specific details of a situation as the client describes it. If in doubt about what the client is describing or explaining, it is important to ask for more detail rather than falling back on assumptions. This is illustrated by Mrs Kennedy's attributions about her husband's memory difficulties. She had been married to her husband for over forty years, he had developed dementia and she became his primary caregiver. Unfortunately, the relationship between Mrs Kennedy and her husband, Ronald, was cold and distant and had been so for many years. Ronald was forgetful and frequently asked the same question over and again. Repetitious questioning made Mrs Kennedy extremely frustrated, and she became quite angry when the same question was asked repeatedly.

Some therapists might make the assumption that anger is an understandable reaction by Mrs Kennedy, and the result of frustration. However, when exploring the reason that Mrs Kennedy became so incensed by repetitious questioning a new understanding was reached. When the therapist asked what it was about the repeated questions that made Mrs Kennedy so angry, she replied: 'he is just asking me this to wind me up, he's doing this to make me lose my cool'. The therapist sought to explore alternative explanations for Ronald asking the same question repeatedly, but only after careful consideration of alternatives was Mrs Kennedy able to consider that her husband's dementia may cause him to forget that he had already asked the question and that it was a function of his increased vulnerability rather than a manifestation of old habits. Using Socratic questioning, and adopting an assumption-free approach, Ronald's behaviour was stripped of its attributed malcontent.

6. Out-of-Session Tasks: Homework

Homework Guidelines

Homework is an essential element of CBT that relies upon a particular mechanism for change called *collaborative empiricism*. Collaborative empiricism may appear to be a confusing term, but it simply means that therapist and client collaborate as equal partners in order that improvement in symptoms is achieved as efficiently as possible. In practice, collaborative empiricism means agreeing on targets within sessions and taking discussion forward in a productive manner so that useful gains in knowledge, skills or problem resolution are achieved. Empiricism here simply means testing things out. Thus, when client and therapist *collaboratively* devise a behavioural experiment as a homework task it should be something that will shed new light on an existing problem, and it should not be readily apparent what the outcome will be. This sometimes makes therapists anxious, as they fear unanticipated consequences and worry that the client may fail in the task or may experience a negative outcome. However, unless something different is tried one will not get different results, and in not taking a risk it is likely that progress towards a positive outcome in therapy will be reduced.

Homework is not an optional extra to be used as and when it suits, but must form part of the start and end of every therapy session, as homework contributes to a better treatment outcome (Coon & Gallagher-Thompson, 2002; Kazantzis et al., 2005).

Therapists exercise control in homework compliance primarily in the assignment of the task, and therefore great care must be taken when negotiating with the client about plans for homework (Tompkins, 2002). In some cases, setting homework can be a challenge for both the therapist and the patient, either because the client finds it difficult to complete the tasks or because the therapist fears the patient will not comply with the homework exercise. It is helpful to review the attributions the client is making about your expectations of them in completing a homework task. In this case, setting up homework as a no-lose experiment can be very productive.

Sometimes the therapist is concerned that their client is physically unable to engage in homework. This is the time to engage in behavioural experiments, set up as no-lose experiments, to ascertain what people can achieve. What a person can achieve when they have motivation and a clear understanding of the rationale for engaging in a homework task can be eye opening for a therapist. In this way, homework can be an education for the therapist as much for the client.

Unless we ask our clients to do something different outside the confines of the therapy clinic, it is hard to see change happening. Homework becomes the test bed for ideas discussed within the session.

Homework should arise from discussions within the session and not be pre-fabricated (therefore you may actually decide upon a homework task midway through the session). You might say to your client: 'what do you think would be a good way to take our discussion further?' as a way of collaboratively agreeing upon a homework task.

Homework should be personally important and relevant to the individual. It should take topics further. It is central to the presenting problems.

Start small and focus on behavioural tasks at first. Asking your client to record aspects of their daily life may be very helpful in socialising them into behaviour monitoring and it provides you with a great deal of data in the session. Remember that there is a danger of building in failure rather than success if you go too fast with tasks – this is often the experience that has brought your client into therapy in the first place.

Homework should be manageable, time-limited and linked to current concerns. Do not ask someone to do something you would be unwilling to do yourself.

Homework should be specific. You and your client should be clear about what is to be done and the reason for agreeing upon this. You might ask your client whether they understand this: 'what is the reason for doing this, what do you think you might gain?'

Homework should be realistic. You might try to help your client problem-solve in advance: 'are there any problems you foresee which might make this task difficult for you to complete?'

Homework is a learning process. It is not necessary that the client has to do everything successfully. The purpose of homework is to find out more about the levels of difficulties experienced by your client. If things do not work out as predicted then a lot can be learned from this experience. Try to set tasks as a no-lose situation. Even if the person has not completed their homework this can be used as a fruitful topic for discussion within session.

Be creative. Take calculated risks when the client is used to doing homework. Note that this does not mean asking your client to do something that is physically dangerous. You should not necessarily be able to know the outcome in advance. Sometimes it can be useful to simply ask your client to 'surprise yourself between now and our next appointment'.

Homework is based upon agreement and collaboration. It is always good practice to work with the client prior to leaving the clinic room in order to try and identify any potential obstacles to the successful completion of homework. It is always a good idea to double check that you have the agreement of the client.

(Laidlaw & Thompson, 2008)

Homework in Practice: Case Example

You may recall Jennifer completing her 'hot cross bun' in an earlier example linked to her perception of being a failure and a poor-decision-maker after having her dog 'rehomed' (see pp. 69–70), Jennifer was asked to complete a homework task about her reasons for having her dog rehoused. The reasons she listed are presented in Table 5.1. In the example here Jennifer is able to see that she has *not* made a mess of things, but has instead found her dog a good home with a younger owner who wanted an energetic dog.

In this case the homework task contributes to Jennifer becoming her own therapist, as it provides disconfirming evidence that she makes poor decisions. By the time this task is completed Jennifer is able to see that her thinking is not always factual and not always helpful to her self-confidence.

Increasing Compliance in Homework Completion

If homework is poorly complied with in therapy, this may be because it is poorly conceptualised and contextualised with the client by the therapist. Therapists who leave the discussion of homework assignment to the last few minutes of a treatment session may find more problems with its execution, as all too frequently homework tasks need to be talked about sufficiently for the client to understand what is being asked of them and how this is linked to their primary presenting problem. You should get into the habit of discussing homework at any time during the session, when it naturally arises as a topic. Garbled instructions with limited time to explain the point of the exercise is not likely to bring about positive results. Any task that fails to establish face-validity will have limited apparent relevance to a resolution of problems as a client sees it, and compliance will be an issue.

Therapists should not underestimate how stressful an incomplete understanding in therapy can be. Without stereotyping older people, it is the experience of this author

TABLE 5.1   *Homework as disconfirming evidence and new understanding*

Reasons for Dasher (dog) to be rehoused

1. Needs a lot of exercise – more that I can give him
2. Dasher has run away and is unpredictable
3. Long-term prospect of his care
4. How I would cope with him, for example with knee replacement?
5. Ball obsession is very wearing
6. Has to be walked even in bad weather
7. Set alarm clock for 3.20 a.m. to let him out
8. Keeping him back, i.e. he needs to run free and play with young people/dogs
9. Can't cope with responsibility of Dasher anymore
10. Uncertainty of him fighting with other dogs
11. Fought with large cream Labrador over ball in semi darkness in the local park
12. Had to leave lunch early to come home for Dasher
13. Curtails freedom
14. Got into panic when I met two large puppies when Dasher had his ball
15. Have no joy in walking him – mostly nervous
16. After a discussion with L (dog handler) about dog walker owners/walking Dasher, I don't feel quite so bad about my own fears – even her own mother has terrible experiences sometimes when walking their own dogs

that older people in the main tend to complete homework diligently, and even when completing homework they are anxious about having done a 'good job'. An older client returning to therapy sessions without having completed their assignment is very stressful and may cause problems in achieving good therapy engagement. For many older clients who were used to being competent and diligent individuals in their previous lives, this failure to apprehend and complete a task may be demoralising – especially as it is a frequent wish of clients that they are seen in a positive light by their therapist, but are often concerned that they are 'too old to learn therapy'.

If the therapist is curious about the outcome of homework, and transmits this curiosity with an appropriate measure of enthusiasm and reinforcement, then homework completion may be more likely (Tompkins, 2002). It is much more likely that homework will be complied with if it is always the first item to be discussed in session after agreeing the agenda.

Other aspects of homework planning that can enhance compliance is to consider role-playing aspects of the homework in session before the client leaves. You are advised to review your conceptualisation diagram with your client at this point to look again at repeated patterns of behaviour. This can be very useful if your client is taking the step of initiating contact with a friend or family member, is asking something of someone or is being assertive. It can be very helpful for the client if you play the role of the family member, and after completing the role play you ascertain how similar the situation feels to real life and how they felt when asserting themselves or asking for help. In addition, it can be useful to add an element to the homework in which the client uses positive self-talk and tries to predict the outcome prior to engaging in the task. This added 'cognitive' element to a behavioural homework task can help a person gain a lot of personally meaningful disconfirmatory evidence.

Another useful task to enhance treatment compliance is to problem solve the completion of homework in advance. Some clients are very keen to get a task done and may be overly optimistic about their ability to complete the task. The therapist needs to make a quick assessment here. If the task is so easy for the client to complete, how is it that they find themselves in your clinic? Thus, take some time to tease out how the client plans to approach the completion of the homework. Do they have a certain day and time to complete this? What obstacles can they foresee?

Increasing Therapeutic Gains from Homework Completion: Putting the C After the B in CBT

It is good practice to see the completion of the task as an opportunity for further learning in the session – completion of homework is not the end of the task. In this way, the therapist devotes a set amount of time to discuss the homework further within the session, with the view that the client learns more from completion of the task, and for the therapist to gain an enhanced understanding of their client. This is seen most clearly when the therapist asks the client to talk about how they feel they have performed in the task and what they may have gained from it.

Anxious clients in particular downgrade their performance and fail to give themselves credit for having completing a task that previously was difficult for them, thus negating any sense of achievement. For example, as part of a wider treatment plan Alice was asked to overcome her anxiety at using her cash card at a bank automatic teller machine. She successfully completed the task. When her therapist asked her to appraise her performance she could not see what her achievements were:

- When asked if she felt a sense of achievement she said: 'No' and 'I feel so stupid'.
- The therapist said: 'let's put this into context, when was the last time you did this on your own? Is there any part of you that deserves some praise?'

In this exchange, the therapist helped the client to think back to how they felt prior to completion of the task, and via Socratic dialogue asked the client to review their fear in advance of the task. The therapist asked the client when she last took money out of a cash machine (she had never done this), and what she would say to someone she was close to in similar circumstances. She was very warm and encouraging, and recognised the level of anxiety the person would need to overcome to complete this task. The therapist encouraged the client to apply this message to herself. Alice said:

- 'It gives me a lift … I didn't run away or avoid it. I did it by myself. I wanted to prove to myself that I'm not frightened'.

From this exchange it should be apparent that a predominantly behavioural task can be enhanced for its learning opportunities by using cognitive skills in CBT. The client can gain so much more when the therapist puts the C after the B in CBT.

Structure in Therapy: Four Treatment Phases in CBT with Older People

CBT is a brief form of psychotherapy, and while the primary aim of CBT is symptom reduction this does not mean that the therapist stays with the client until they are cured of all symptoms. Rather, when a client has the skills and competence to manage their problems by themselves, treatment can end. A typical treatment package of CBT often lasts for 16–20 sessions with three distinct phases: early, middle and late.

Early Phase of Treatment (Session 1 to Session 6)

By the end of the first phase of treatment you will have established a good therapeutic relationship and may have contracted to meet for more sessions after a review. In the early phase of treatment clients are socialised into the cognitive model, and are educated about the process of therapy and the nature of depression or anxiety as it impacts on the individual.

It is often helpful and reassuring to the client if the therapist agrees to review therapy goals and progress periodically throughout treatment. It is during this phase of treatment that the therapist may be working hard to establish a *therapeutic relationship*. It is also important that the therapist keeps to the idea that he/she is there to act as a coach and not as an expert or guru who can 'fix' the client's problems. Rather, CBT works best when therapist and client work together by combining their joint expertise – thus the client is the expert on their problems and the way they see the world, while the therapist is the expert in a type of practical therapy and in understanding depression and anxiety in a more general sense.

In the beginning of treatment with CBT it is vital to set out goals for treatment so as to establish a focus for working collaboratively, but also to set down criteria for when treatment will end. Usually, goal setting can be achieved by the end of the third session, although in some cases it may have been achieved much earlier. To achieve a set of goals it is necessary, with your client, to work out what they see as their main problems or difficulties, and to translate their problem list into a goal list to work towards.

It is important to socialise the client into the process of therapy from the first minute of the first session, and as such agreeing goals can be an important task. As you start treatment it is essential that you are clear about what symptoms you are aiming to reduce and how your focus fits with the problems experienced by your client.

Aims for Early Phase of CBT

By the end of the first phase of CBT treatment you ought to have:

- Identified main problem(s) with client and translated this into an agreed goal list to work towards
- Established a strong therapeutic alliance in order to bring about change
- Socialised your client to the cognitive model and the structure of sessions, and established the importance of homework as a treatment component
- Introduced targeted psychoeducation, measurement and self-monitoring as important treatment elements
- Started to develop a case conceptualisation or formulation that you can share with your client

Middle Phase of CBT Treatment

The middle phase of therapy is where the bulk of the work is done and the therapist draws upon the full range of cognitive and behavioural techniques. It is also the time when homework tasks are transformed from data gathering exercises to ways in which the individual experiments with change, and as such can be quite complex and emotive. The middle phase may also see a revision to previous conceptualisations that have been shared with the client as new understandings are reached. In the middle phase of treatment, a decision will be reached as to whether it is necessary to engage in schema change work. During the middle phase of treatment, the goals of treatment may be renegotiated. It is also at this time that the end of therapy will become evident, as change starts to take hold and the client may wish to discuss possible options as they move closer to the end of treatment.

During the middle phase of treatment the client may wonder about what progress they are making. Depressed clients will have a tendency to negatively evaluate progress and anxious clients will worry that insufficient progress has been made to this point, and they may be inclined to push forward towards goals in a self-defeating way that can be very challenging for therapists to deal with. Sooner or later your client will want to ask you how you think they are doing in therapy. The therapist who answers this question with a question – 'how well do you think you are doing?' – may find interesting answers, but fails to address your client's important questions.

Mr Holman was concerned that he wasn't making enough progress in therapy and was thinking of discontinuing treatment. The therapist has at least three options:

1. Agree that he should discontinue sessions, as his feelings about progress are probably right
2. Tell him not to worry, and say that he is making good progress
3. Take time in the session to discuss the evidence for and against his thoughts

When thinking about these the three possible actions you may consider the following:

1. This is an example of emotional reasoning (I feel anxious therefore it must be right that I'm not doing well) and a good opportunity for some quick psychoeducation of your client and possible thought monitoring
2. This is reassurance giving, and very likely to be repeated at every session unless you can help the client find an answer that they can give themselves
3. This is an example of collaborative empiricism in action, and therefore the correct thing to do

There is value in all three options, but being collaborative and empirical means taking option 3.

What the therapist did was compare current to previous weekly activity diaries and show Mr Holman that he was now doing more activities than at the start of therapy. He had increased his attendance at his local gym and he had also taken part in a number of social events that previously he had avoided. He had also resumed playing the piano. This approach used collaborative empiricism as it utilised the evidence to address his fears. It is helpful to remember that people who are depressed make many cognitive errors, and that these can also relate to perceived progress in therapy. Here, the personal data provided by the client becomes powerful answers as well as powerful learning opportunities. Often clients get frustrated by having to record thoughts or activities in diaries, but an example of their use as a tool to assess change can make measurement seem integral to treatment.

Aims for Middle Phase of CBT

By the end of the middle phase of CBT treatment you ought to have:

- Shared a case conceptualisation and perhaps revised conceptualisation
- Taught your client how behaviour and mood are linked via activity monitoring

- Introduced problem-solving techniques
- Introduced behaviour experiments to challenge previously held beliefs
- Introduced thought monitoring and cognitive restructuring
- Introduced resilience- and compassion-based approaches that are age-specific and acknowledge the skills level of the client
- Decided whether to adopt schema change techniques

Final Phase of Treatment

In the final phase of therapy, two main tasks remain to be accomplished: (1) the agreement of an appropriate termination point for therapy; and (2) the elaboration of a relapse prevention plan.

Depending upon the service you work in, or the role you occupy, you may not have as many degrees of freedom when it comes to modifying the end of treatment. Regardless, you will want to attempt to achieve a good ending with your client so that they have a sense of control over how therapy ends.

While it is not always possible to have a good ending, or you may need to agree an ending with a client as they have not achieved sufficient progress, you will still want to ensure that this is done in tandem with the client's wishes where possible. In such cases, the therapist will work with the client to agree possible options and make arrangements for follow-on treatment before therapy ends. The appropriate task is to try to ensure the client has a role in deciding the next steps, and that a negative sense of failure is not internalised by the client. Equally, the responsibility for the therapy not working should not be personalised.

It is simply the case that not all therapies are suitable to every client, and sometimes the timings for interventions and therapy are not optimal. It is important for the client's possible future engagement with psychotherapy that they do not feel they have failed.

Jakobsons et al. (2007) have identified seven criteria that guide the decision as to whether therapists have reached the point at which the client can be discharged from therapy. The box-out below shows the seven criteria. See how many you can tick when thinking about a specific client with whom you have reached the point at which to discontinue therapy. The seven criteria are challenging to meet in their entirety for every client.

Seven criteria for when therapy should end:

- Decrease in symptoms measured by psychometrically robust scale
- Decrease of symptoms is stable and maintained for at least eight weeks
- Decrease in functional impairment is evident

(Continued)

(Continued)

- Decrease in symptoms is not temporary
- Evidence of spontaneous use of new skills at time of stress
- Sense of pride in use of new skills in contrast to patient doubt of the utility of techniques, skills or coping resources
- Evidence of generalisation linked with symptom decrease elsewhere

(Jakobsons et al., 2007)

Endings in CBT have often been minimised because of the de-emphasis of the importance of the therapist–client relationship (Ochoa & Muran, 2008). It can be important to allow the client to have as much input into the ending as is possible once the final number of sessions has been agreed.

Michael was seen by his therapist for a long time as he had experienced a number of loss experiences and age-related challenges that had changed the emphasis and goals for therapy. When discharge was agreed and set, Michael completed a relapse prevention task, but also wrote a more personal 'end of term report' that outlined what he had gained in therapy and what he would miss. This is reproduced here:

'Never too close [professional boundaries], but an ear to listen and be positive, never undermining, always debating, and finding alternatives, never criticising. Most of all the opportunity to talk and debate to an agenda that was always stimulating and intelligent.'

For Michael it was part of the collaboration of therapy between himself and his therapist that he should be able to have a say in how treatment ended. This was also an opportunity for him to be able to say what he would miss, and for this to be discussed openly and honestly in therapy before it ended.

Termination is an issue identified at the start of therapy as evidenced by the need to establish goals early on. 'CBT ends when the goals of therapy identified at the beginning of treatment are met, and the patient has acquired the tools by which to function as his or her own therapist when future difficulties arise' (Ochoa & Muran, 2008: 201).

Prior to termination of treatment, it can be helpful to engage the client in a review of what they have learned from therapy, listing what strategies have worked well. This task is very useful as a self-review homework task. Let's return to Jennifer, who we met at the start of this chapter when she was just starting therapy. By the end of therapy her therapist suggested she work on a list that outlined what she had learned from therapy and how she may deal with any future lapses or challenges. Table 5.2 reproduces Jennifer's list.

As you can see from Jennifer's list, she has identified quite a few positives that she has gained in her time in therapy (her BDI scores also fell markedly from baseline). Most of these 'gains' are personal to her and the work she did in therapy, and it should be obvious that any relapse prevention guide has to be individualised and cannot be pre-manufactured or directed by the therapist. It is important to assist your client in thinking about how to apply their gains.

TABLE 5.2   *Jennifer's list*

Make a list of what you have gained from us working together

1. Try not to panic
2. Learning from my own experiences
3. Using those experiences in times of stress
4. Search 'inwards' instead of 'outside' [for answers] during stressful periods
5. 'I do matter' – believe in myself
6. 'I can do this' – tackle problems and win
7. There are always two sides to a coin – you have taught me to think problems through and try to work them out for myself

What could you use to help yourself in future?

I could use the problems which I have experienced through my life to help me deal with stressful periods which may occur in the present or future.

Money-Back Guarantees?

For some clients it is especially helpful for them to have a sense that they can get back in touch should there be a crisis or event that requires input. If you are in a position to offer it, it may be helpful for the client to be able to contact you directly if they feel they require a booster session. In my own clinical practice, I have offered clients a 'six-month guarantee'. I often make a joke about not buying shoes without some sort of guarantee for workmanship. Thus, if clients feel that their problems recur or have not sufficiently resolved I am happy to have them come right back to me within six months of the end of therapy. Very few clients have ever needed to invoke my poor workmanship guarantee, but while it is impossible to say this with scientific precision, my impression is that most clients leave therapy reassured and with a sense of connection.

Relapse prevention helps the client to identify and anticipate potential challenging situations that may trigger a relapse (Overholser, 1998). As a relapse is unlikely to result from a single situation, the therapist works with the client to anticipate how they might respond to certain stressors and to imagine possible strategies they may employ to help them manage. It may be helpful to role play some of the identifiable challenges with the person prior to discharge. When role playing, the therapist should take on the role of the client and the client can either act as the therapist or as a person being challenging to them in imagined stressful situations. It can be helpful for the client to see relapse prevention as an opportunity to apply their problem-solving skills learned in therapy, especially if this is done with positive and supportive feedback on the client's performance. It can also be a good opportunity to help the client set realistic expectations for themselves outside of the therapy session. Life is never without its ups and downs, and clients can experience challenging situations that do not necessarily indicate a return of their symptoms. Overholser (1995, 1998) suggests using the term 'lapse' to promote realistic expectations.

Fourth Phase in a Three-Phase Model of CBT!

As it sometimes happens that older people who attend therapy for depression or anxiety may have other physical health problems, or who may confront some age-related challenge, therapy can extend beyond a 16–20 session format. This may mean that endings in therapy can become more challenging, for therapist and the client. Thus, it may be useful to take a different approach to endings with clients in this case. It may be efficient and more productive to reduce contact before discharge (booster sessions) and to offer a way back if there is a relapse.

Using Booster Sessions Prior to Discharge

At the end of treatment, intermittent or booster sessions can be agreed upon in advance of discharge. This can be very helpful, especially if you have worked with your client for a prolonged period of time, or when you and your client have established an especially strong therapeutic bond. Endings may be the wrong way to think about it in CBT. For the client this is the start of a new phase. This 'next phase' of treatment is a transitional one, and like all transitions it can be anxiety-provoking at the start but confidence-building in the end. Thus, when working with your client allow a discussion about what they might miss about attending therapy, but also discuss what they might gain from therapy ending at this point. Placed in a developmental frame of reference, the end of therapy is not the end but the start of the next natural phase in which they can become their own therapists. The aim in CBT is to help people become their own therapists, so we should be sorry to see the person go but glad they have 'graduated'.

Aims for the Final Phase of CBT

By the end of the final phase of CBT treatment you ought to have:

- Agreed an appropriate end point for therapy that is a positive step forward on a journey your client will complete by themselves
- Acknowledged the strength and resilience of your client
- Acknowledged that saying goodbye is hard and it is not unusual for clients to feel anxious at the end of treatment
- Encouraged your client to create their own relapse prevention plan from a review of what they have gained by working with you

Summary

CBT has a unique format for helping the client to empower themselves by taking personal responsibility for change. The therapist cannot change people but can work with their client to support them in challenging the status quo. However, get the structure right and therapy becomes a less complex scenario for clients. If you use the structure and excel in it, it will empower you to become a better therapist.

Learning Log: Reflection and Review

- Think of a recent session you completed. What aspects of the structure of CBT did you find the most challenging to use?
- In terms of continuing to improve your application of CBT in practice, use a copy of the CTS-R (see www.get.gg/docs/CTSR.pdf) and rate yourself on each of the domains. Be kind but realistic. Focus on areas where you feel you are weakest. Make an action plan to address some areas of your practice.
- Ask one of your clients for permission to tape a session and discuss your CTS-R rating with your supervisor.

Further Reading

The following sources provide more in-depth coverage of topics raised in this chapter.

Beck, J. S. (2011). *Cognitive behavior therapy: basics and beyond* (2nd ed.). New York: Guilford Press.

Blackburn, I. M., James, I. A., Milne, D. L., Baker, C., Standart, S., Garland, A., & Reichelt, F. K. (2001). The revised cognitive therapy scale (CTS-R): psychometric properties. *Behavioural and Cognitive Psychotherapy, 29,* 431–446.

Kazantzis, N., Deane, F. R., Ronan, K. R., & L'Abate, L. (2005). *Using homework assignments in cognitive behavior therapy.* New York: Routledge.

Six

The Therapeutic Relationship in CBT with Older People

Learning Objectives
By the end of this chapter you will:

- Learn how working with older people may have unique features and unique challenges
- Become familiar with the concept of cohort factors in therapy and understand how to become insightful about generational differences
- Understand the importance of common and non-common factors in psychotherapy
- Identify the key components of a good working alliance
- Apprehend and apply pro-social behaviours in therapy, which promote a collaborative and trusting working alliance that empowers clients and facilitates clinical change

Introduction: Working with Older People in Therapy

Chronological age provides limited data by itself, so therapists working with older people need to spend time understanding the appropriate developmental context in which a person may experience depression or anxiety disorders. There can be specific issues in working with older people that are different from working age adults: 'While the models used for general adults are often useful for [use with] elders they are also incomplete in defining the complexities that are especially relevant to clinical interventions for the elderly (Sadavoy, 2009: 810).

Sadavoy (2009) provides some guidance for therapists working with older clients when he proposes five 'C's' associated with psychogeriatrics: chronicity, complexity, comorbidity, continuity and context. The suggestions by Sadavoy (2009) acknowledge that working with older people can be challenging. Continuity refers to the fact that older people bring the product of their past experiences and beliefs into the current experience. This may result in clients having different capacities and abilities that may impact upon the therapeutic relationship. Thus, the therapist may need to understand the lifespan continuity of the client in terms of its impact upon their ability to be understood and to trust. When listening to the client talk about their life experiences the therapist needs to listen for any potential therapeutic alliance ruptures that result. The context of working with older people may be understood by reference to the social, environmental and physical contexts in which the client interacts and impacts upon. Anxiety and depression can be better understood by taking account of the client's context. Clearly context and continuity factors need to be taken into account in the early sessions of CBT in order that your therapeutic relationship is strengthened by the increased sense your client will gain of being understood. The therapist needs to be flexible in responding authentically and flexibly to the client, to work within their worldview, in order to produce a working relationship (Dryden, 2009). Some clients may want a friendly/informal therapist and others may want a knowledgeable/containing 'expert'. The trick is for the therapist to remain collaborative and in synch with the client.

As CBT promotes an empirical approach to psychological therapy, sessions and treatment packages with the client are likely to be highly structured. It requires attention by the therapist to ensure that structure does not engender passivity or dependence in the client. Older people may be especially prone to becoming passive in their interactions with you, as they will have been socialised into working with healthcare professionals at a time when there was a different approach to care. It is important that the client feel able to trust you and yet at the same time feel that you retain a strong professional code of conduct. If we are to expect our clients to share their thoughts, emotions and actions with us, especially at a time when they may be feeling exceptionally vulnerable or when their actions are viewed through a personal lens of shame and guilt, then we need to work hard to establish a good trusting relationship by the end of the second session.

Collaboration is emphasised in CBT and occurs when the client and their therapist work together to develop a respectful dyadic relationship that recognises each other's strengths and draws on the separate competences to bring about meaningful and lasting change. An important product of a collaborative therapeutic relationship in CBT will be a strong therapeutic alliance. This is when the two partners in the dyad agree a common set of goals to deal with an agreed set of problems.

The Therapeutic Relationship in CBT

When practising CBT, we ought to pay special attention to the development of a strong working relationship with our clients, but this by itself is unlikely to be sufficient to bring about good treatment outcomes (Dryden, 2009), as this is considered *necessary but not sufficient* (Beck et al., 1979: 45) within CBT.

The therapeutic relationship in CBT is important as a means of promoting change and helping individuals to overcome difficulties, as in therapy we often require our clients to talk to us about behaviours, thoughts and feelings that our clients would not normally discuss, and in some cases would prefer to keep hidden. However, a psychological therapy treatment package for depression and anxiety means working with people when they feel especially emotionally vulnerable. Hence our relationship and the trust we engender is going to be important in determining how far our clients are willing to challenge themselves towards growth (Dryden & Branch, 2012).

Essential to achieving a good outcome in CBT is achieving a collaborative working alliance, and most likely this is formed very early on in treatment and may occur as soon as the first session. Nelson and Politano (1993: 255) note the importance of the therapeutic relationship across the whole treatment 'package' in CBT, affecting every stage of treatment from start to finish, and that this requires therapists to be active in understanding:

> How the therapeutic relationship effects cooperation, truthful feedback from the client, therapist as model, etc., and how this then influences the client's perspective of self-efficacy, benefits of therapy, etc., all of which can interactively impact on generalization and maintenance of therapeutic gains.

CBT is an active and directive treatment approach, which means that the therapist will introduce clients to a new set of skills that they can use to deal with their presenting problems. It is directive in that the therapist ensures that attention is directed to the resolution of problems, and active in that the client is expected to be an active participant in their own treatment package.

Thus, the development of a working alliance can occur through the therapist using the nature of the relationship to promote change by observing in-session behaviours that may indicate how the client operates outside of therapy and which may cause them problems. As Safran and Segal (1996: 37) note:

> Because cognitive therapy concerns itself explicitly with understanding and modifying perceptions, there is certainly no reason, in theory, for cognitive therapists to avoid investigating the relationship between patient's perceptions and the therapeutic alliance. To do this however, requires an understanding of the patient's characteristic way of construing events by identifying both the specific, interpersonal patterns that tend to be linked to this construal style and the events that take place in the therapeutic interaction.

Who are You?

Let's think about you! Are there some people you have found it easier to be with? In some situations in your life perhaps you have sought friendships (alliances) with certain types of individuals. If you have ever been in a crisis, what types of people did you turn to for advice? What are the characteristics that you have sought out (i.e. what makes you turn to them)? What does this say about you as a person? Maybe you also wish to reflect on what behaviours you express when you feel vulnerable? This may only be a small aspect of your overall characteristics, but would you wish to be judged on this alone?

Maybe this exercise will give you some idea of the types of helpful behaviours you could to display and model for your client as you seek to build a helpful and helping relationship with them.

Make some notes here.

Working with Older People in Therapy: Relationship Factors

Age Differences Between Therapist and Client

When working with older clients it can be important to ascertain how they wish to be addressed during therapy. Never assume, as you attempt to relax your client into an informal working relationship with you, that using first names will be acceptable. It is always better to adopt a more formal respectful addressing of the client until you are invited to use their first name.

The therapist may be up to five or six decades younger than their client. Just as you are open-minded about what you expect your client to achieve in your sessions together, and you do not expect your client to be treated to an ageist perspective, you also do not need to apologise for your own age. It can be an asset that you and the client come from different generations – if you both appreciate and value the differences in perspective this may promote an interesting dialogue when it comes to understanding situations. You may wish to have a brief discussion about whether the age difference between you will be a factor to consider when working together. This brief discussion within the first phase of therapy can promote greater understanding between therapist and client. It can be done very respectfully by the therapist, who may explain that as they were born at a different time from the client, it might be useful for the therapist to figure out what values they have that may be influenced by their upbringing. It also provides the therapist with an opportunity to mention that they respect the life experience the client has. This can also lead into a discussion about the influence of cohort beliefs.

Cohort Factors

Cohort can be understood simply as values and beliefs shared among a generational group of individuals born at a similar time period. Taking account of cohort beliefs, allows a therapist to acknowledge that different generations have different experiences that shape their values and world view and as such these may have changed across generations. Knight (2006) notes working with older people entails learning something of the folkways of people born many years before.

Example of Cohort Transmission of Beliefs at a Personal Level

In order for therapist to reflect on the importance of cohort beliefs and values, consider the current cohort of older people who are true age pioneers as they tend to live much longer than their parents and grandparents and may do so in a healthier state. Consider an 82-year-old woman alive today. Born in 1932, her own father was born in 1901 when life expectancy at birth in the UK was 45 for men. Her grandparents were born in the nineteenth century and would likely have been born between 1870 and 1880. Octogenarian clients in your clinic therefore have models of ageing drawn from grandparents alive during the Victorian era, and therapists are communicating across a number of generations that are completely different from their own experience. Importantly, clients born in the 1920s and 1930s have a very different experience from therapists in that they have lived in a time before the NHS and universal coverage. These clients have known a time when there was no social welfare and may have experienced poverty unknown in the time of therapists. Thus, the current cohort of older people may influence the values of clients in ways that may be very different from the experience of the therapist.

Generational Cohorts

The baby boomers (born from 1945 to 1961) are an example of a cohort, as they are conventionally believed to adopt similar outlooks and values. The baby boomers were all born in the post-World War II baby boom era, hence their name, and have witnessed great social change over their lifetime.

The baby boomers can be split into different cohorts: 'leading edge', born between 1946 and 1955; and 'later born', born between 1956 and 1961. The 'leading edge' baby boomers experienced and contributed to the social upheavals of the 1960s. On average, baby boomers tend to be better educated, more ethnically diverse and more likely to be divorced or separated with fewer children than previous generations (Pruchno, 2012). For an interesting positive exploration of baby boomers, visit: www.aarp.org/personal-growth/transitions/boomers_65 and for revisionist views see www.huffingtonpost.com/renee-fisher/baby-boomers_b_4445742.html

Baby Boomers?

The baby boomers were all born in the post-World War II baby boom, hence their name. Usually they are the generation born between 1945 and 1961.

They're Here!

By 2011 the first baby boomers had reached retirement age (Pruchno, 2012).

> ## Agents of Change?
>
> The early born cohort (leading edge baby boomers representing half of this generational cohort) in this generation grew up during the 1960s and brought about a lot of social change by rejecting 'traditional' values and social norms. The phrase 'baby boomer' is used as a cultural description as much as a demographic one.

More usually, age cohorts can be located by generational groups such as those in their 60s (born in the 1950s), 70s (born in the 1940s) and 80 or older (born in the 1920s and 1930s). It may help you get a sense of what the different generations have experienced by looking at Table 6.1.

From Table 6.1, one can see that each generational cohort had deprivations and sacrifices that would have resulted in consequences for family life. As a result, many older people find it hard to tolerate waste of food and find themselves affected by family stories and experiences of real hardship and poverty. Most of today's therapists working with older people will be part of the UK generation that never fought in a major war, and most people born in 1960 onwards did not experience conscription. The notable events in the history of the UK often have personal resonances to the clients you will work with, and becoming knowledgeable about some aspects of these events may help you to understand your client in a more elaborated context.

Cohort Beliefs and Therapy Process

While cohort beliefs suggest that in some cases the therapist's values may not entirely align with older people because of being born and having lived in different social milieu, especially when the age difference between therapist and client is more than three or four decades, the therapist may find it useful to learn something of the social history of the country or culture of the population they work with.

One needs to be aware that these differences may interfere with the establishment of a solid working relationship. An example of where social history may educate you about some of the mores and attitudes of your clients when they were younger is illustrated by the tragic case of Alan Turing. Turing was a brilliant mathematician largely credited with breaking the enigma code during World War II, and his achievements undoubtedly shortened the war and saved countless lives. Yet he was treated abysmally when he was discovered to be homosexual (he was convicted of 'gross indecency' in 1952). He endured androgenic injections (chemical castration) before taking his own life in 1954. In 2009, Prime Minister Gordon Brown recognised Alan Turing's contributions to the war effort and his pioneering and brilliant advances in computing (he is considered by many as the father of modern computing) and issued a formal government apology. Gordon Brown said this: 'While Turing was dealt with under the law of the time ... his treatment was of course utterly unfair, and I am pleased to have the chance to say how deeply sorry I and we all are for what happened to him.' As a postscript to this story, on Christmas Eve 2013,

TABLE 6.1 *Cohort experiences: major life events for generations born between 1930 and 1960*

People born 1920–1939 **People born in the 1920s are in their 90s now**	• In 1920 in the US women gain the right to vote (in the UK this happened in 1918). • In 1920 Oxford University admits its first woman undergraduate. • In 1922 the BBC begins broadcasting. • In 1926 the UK experiences a general strike. • In 1928 penicillin is discovered by Alexander Fleming, revolutionising medical survival rates. • In 1929 the great financial crash results in a long-lasting and deep economic recession with high levels of unemployment and poverty. • Driving tests and speed limits introduced in Britain in 1934. • Jarrow march takes place in 1936 as men march for the right to work. • In 1939 World War II begins, plunging 'victorious' Britain into a major role change within the global context – no longer a world power.
People born 1940–1949 **People born in the 1940s are in their 70s now**	• 1940 – Battle of Britain with the RAF fighting to repel invasion. Britain holds it breathe for invasion. Major cities experience Blitz. • In 1940 food rationing is introduced to the UK. In 1948 flour rationing ends and in 1949 clothes rationing ends, but some rationing continues into the early 1950s (sweets, soap, tea). It took until 1958 for rationing of coal to end. • 1945 – war ends but attrition and austerity continues until the end of the decade. Make do and mend is a way of life for many. • In 1948 the NHS is born and universal free healthcare becomes a reality for people. • In 1948 the WHO is founded by the United Nations, itself founded in 1945.
People born 1950–1960 **People born in the 1950s are in their 60s now**	• First non-stop transatlantic flights introduced in 1950. • In 1950 the Korean War draws the UK and US into another conflict. Many Korean veterans feel forgotten and neglected on their return. • In 1952 the polio vaccine becomes available. • In 1952 Britain carries out its first nuclear bomb tests.

- In 1953 19-year-old Derek Bentley is hanged for his part in the 'murder' of a PC. Later post-humouesly pardoned in 1993.
- In 1955 Ruth Ellis becomes the last woman to be hanged for murder.
- In 1956 the Suez Crisis begins, symbolising Britain's decline as a global power.
- In 1957 the Wolfenden report recommends that homosexual acts in private should no longer be a criminal offence – takes until 1967 to be enacted in law.
- In 1958 the first UK motorway opens (the M1 opens in 1959).
- 1958 coal rationing ends.
- 1960 Penguin wins the right to publish *Lady Chatterley's Lover*. Famously, the prosecutor in the case asked 'Is it a book you would wish your wife or servants to read?' Widely held to be the start of the swinging 60s.

Events important for the baby boomers

- Assassination of John F. Kennedy, Robert F. Kennedy and Martin Luther King.
- Woodstock, Beatlemania.
- The 'pill and the sexual revolution'.
- Equality for women.
- TV in the home. Change to colour TV in early 1970s.
- Internet becomes part of our lives.
- Moon landings, Vietnam war, Watergate, Falklands war, Thatcherism and the miner's strike.

the Queen (Elizabeth II) issued a posthumous Royal Pardon to Alan Turing with regard to his conviction for homosexuality. The Royal Pardon allows people to reflect upon the many injustices visited on so many individuals in the intervening years since the 1950s. You might wish to reflect on how far British society has come in terms of its attitudes and the great social change that has taken place over recent decades – decades that your clients lived through from beginning to end.

Cohort: Hanging on to Secrets of the Past

Working with older people who are gay can sometimes require the therapist to explore how open the person feels they can be with the therapist. Gay older women and men will have faced a lot of hostility and prejudice growing up, and may have experienced direct discrimination because of their sexual orientation. Mr Jonson is 71 years old and is the primary caregiver for his partner who has MS and is wheelchair bound. Mr Jonson is very open about his sexual orientation but when he was a young man in his thirties in the early 1970s he 'came out' to his employer, a local businessman. He was sacked shortly afterwards. Mr Jonson believes it was because his employer was homophobic. Younger therapists working with older gay men and women may wish to reflect that for many this carried quite a stigma. Thus your client may have developed a habit of keeping details back from people for fear of rejection.

When working with older people, therapists need to take account of the stigmatising cohort beliefs that may have existed at the time and be mindful of the importance of building rapport through trust within the relationship in CBT. It can also be the case that older people whose adult children are gay may find this a challenging transition precisely because of cohort beliefs, and because they may have grown up retaining certain beliefs. Although not writing about CBT, Hinrichsen (2010) writes very well on this topic.

Warmth, Empathy, Congruence?

Psychological therapies are made up of common and non-common factors, although common factors are more important in determining the nature of the therapeutic relationship (Hyer et al., 2004). Warmth, genuineness and empathy found in different types of therapeutic approaches regardless of philosophical orientation, are common factors (see Roth & Pilling, 2007) that are used to build a trusting working relationship within therapy. CBT is no different in expecting therapists to adopt certain helpful characteristics as well as developing therapy-specific (i.e. CBT) and problem-specific (i.e. presentation of common mental health problems) competences (Roth & Pilling, 2007).

Common Factors?

- Developing trust
- Achieving empathic understanding

- Displaying warmth, genuineness and acceptance (unconditional positive regard)
- Empowering the client
- Collaboration – therapist adopts role of coach, not expert

Carl Rogers, a noted psychotherapist in the 1950s and 1960s, introduced the idea that unconditional positive regard, comprising explicit valuing, acceptance and non-judgemental trust approaches to the client on the part of the therapist (Kirschenbaum & Henderson, 1990), were essential for change to occur in therapy. Beck et al. (1979), in the classic 'manual' on how to do cognitive therapy, devote a chapter to the therapeutic relationship and emphasise the importance of warmth, accurate empathy and genuineness (so-called common factors) for therapists wishing to build trust and rapport in order to help the client overcome habit and ingrained maladaptive behaviours. Beck et al. (1979: 46) caution that 'Cognitive and behavioural techniques often *seem* deceptively simple. Consequently, the neophyte therapist may become "gimmick-oriented" to the point of ignoring the human aspects of the therapist–patient interaction.'

Alliance-Promoting Behaviours in Therapy: Do More!

Summarising frequently in early sessions to check on understandings.

Giving empathic responses to description of problems, e.g. 'It sounds as if life has not been easy these last few months', 'It's a good step to seek help now, even though this must be very difficult for you.'

Maintaining eye contact and responding to emotional changes in the sessions.

Being consistent, calm and respectful – reacting appropriately when necessary.

Alliance-Damaging Behaviours in Therapy: Do Less!

Having a rushed, inconsistent approach to therapy – seeming unprepared and lacking confidence.

Displaying safety-seeking 'Pandora's box' behaviour – not wanting to ask 'difficult' questions for fear of not being able to handle what comes next.

Using preformed questions and preformed homework tasks – not listening intently to what client says or how things are said.

Failing to give encouragement and praise to client – failing to realise how difficult it may be for the client to engage in therapy.

Older people born in different times from the therapist may hold attitudes and beliefs that differ from those of the therapist, and can damage the development of the therapeutic alliance.

The older male client with 'traditional' values may be seen by a younger female therapist as sexist, or even misogynist, which can create confusion on both sides. The therapist may accept the individual while not accepting their behaviour, not condoning or colluding with behaviour that is considered unethical or antisocial. The therapist ought not to judge, but accept the client has developed their beliefs from a different era. Wilkins (2000) points out that unconditional positive regard is very different from liking the client, – what remains important in establishing a strong therapeutic relationship is the therapist's ability to remain congruent.

For CBT therapists, one of the goals of therapy may be facilitating a change in the way that clients habitually treat themselves, especially in crises. The nature of the therapeutic relationship can be modelled for the client. The client may value your positive orientation towards them, but may find this difficult to internalise and use as a tool for change. The key aim here is for the client to realise that you accept them, not because you are being nice, or because it is expected of your role, but because acceptance can allow you to look at aspects of thoughts, feelings and behaviour free from negative judgements and negative emotions such as guilt or shame.

It is not uncommon for older people to have grown up in an era when times were hard and people were encouraged to be independent, 'to stand on their own two feet' (cohort belief), and this can foster a sense of needing help or support as a character flaw or a sign of weakness. An empathetic, warm therapist will identify this as a problem to be addressed early in therapy, and an effective CBT therapist will use these elements but also see an opportunity to help the client identify belief structures that are unhelpful and undermining in their attempts to overcome their problems.

When a person develops either anxiety or depression, they may become hard on themselves and believe that if they do treat themselves harshly they will cause even more problems for themselves. Being compassionate and caring to oneself does not necessarily come easily to people. Neff and Vonk (2009: 26) note that 'Although people typically value being kind and compassionate to others, they are often harsh and uncaring towards themselves.' This is very true of 70-year-old Michael. He becomes infuriated with himself when he perceives that his memory lets him down. His emotional responses (anger, frustration) to perceived memory failings tend to overwhelm him at a time when he is already distressed. This has increased his sense of incompetence and corroded his view of himself. In therapy, when discussing his latest 'failure', he was asked whether he could try being more accepting of his memory difficulties and more compassionate towards himself so as to reduce his catastrophising. His response was: 'Beating yourself up is a passive process. It's so easy, you fall into that trap so easily. It's such a bloody effort to be compassionate [to oneself] because it's alien. It's not a natural process. It's a struggle [to be compassionate].' After a short pause for reflection, Michael added 'I have lost confidence in my own strengths.'

Therapists need to bear in mind that enabling clients to develop self-acceptance is a skill that may enable them to become their own therapists. In order for clients to develop a more self-compassionate approach within therapy, this behaviour may have to be modelled first by the therapist.

In order for clients to be active participants in their own treatment, a trusting and mutually respectful therapeutic relationships needs to be developed and nurtured. There needs to be some sense of shared ownership for the problem and the resolution of it. Thus psychoeducation about psychological problems and symptoms, as well as about aspects of the therapy itself, will allow your client to become a much more equal participant in treatment.

Humour can be used judiciously in helping a client consider the way they are thinking about things. Done sensitively, the client can see the logical extension of their thoughts, and this can help defuse a potentially stressful situation in therapy. Older people are no different from any other client group in wanting to feel accepted and understood by their therapist. If a client feels that their therapist is consistent, calm and collected, and is approachable and at times light-hearted in defusing intense situations, this can build a strong bond between client and therapist.

As well as humour, CBT therapists tend to be more open in style (Dryden & Branch, 2012), and for older people experiencing the intensity of therapy for the first time it can be comforting getting to know a little bit about their therapist. Many times this author has found himself subjected to questions about family, and while in earlier days I would deflect these questions by suggesting that time within the session was better spent focusing on the client's problems (something that is useful to remind clients as a way of keeping hold of boundaries), it can also be efficient to answer some questions in a low-key, straightforward way before redirecting the client to the session's focus. This type of approach strengthens the sense that you and your client are a team working together to improve outcomes. It strengthens the sense that if *you* will answer questions honestly, your expectation is that the client will also do this. At times when a client has asked a question about family composition (and received an answer), they may sometimes apologise for being too inquisitive. I take the opportunity to say that while the main focus in sessions is the work we have in hand, I know that I ask clients questions all the time with an expectation of honest non-defensive answers, so I will do the same as long as it does not deflect us away from our main focus.

When considering the importance of the therapeutic relationship with older people in CBT, the therapist may wish to take account of age-associated emotional changes (Hyer et al., 2004). Socio-emotional selectivity theory (Carstensen et al., 1999; Carstensen et al., 2003; Scheibe & Carstensen, 2010) suggests that as people age, the perceived finite boundary to their lifespan results in changes to their values so that people preferentially invest in more emotionally meaningful goals, with enhanced emotional regulation as an outcome. Carstensen et al. (2011) have shown that older people are better at emotional regulation and have better emotional stability than adults of working age. Perhaps as people age, life experiences influence how they react to situations, and a more complex emotional competency develops. 'There is no doubt that experience plays a central role in improvements in emotion regulation across the life course, and every reason to think that experience is largely beneficial' (Carstensen et al., 2003: 108). Put more simply, life shaves off the rough edges in our emotional responses and we become less reactive and more proactive. This finds resonance in Carstensen's work, as older people appear to be more skilled at anticipating and therefore avoiding emotionally negative situations, rather than better at dealing with emotionally challenging situations (Scheibe & Carstensen, 2010).

Thus, as older people value emotion regulation and strive to achieve more supportive and nurturing relationships with a smaller circle of significant others (Carstensen et al.,

1999) this suggests benefits for therapists working with older people. In comparison to previous attitudes – that older people would not benefit from psychological therapy – older people may be more emotionally ready for therapy than any other age group. Therefore, a strong therapeutic relationship will be a high priority for your client as well as for you. This is summed up very succinctly by Bob Knight (2006: 24), who notes that:

> The more traditional, largely pessimistic, view has been that adult development and increased experience make people rigid and set in their ways. Yet some clinicians working with the elderly have felt that the effect is quite the reverse: that growth and experience teaches adults to be more flexible, less dogmatic, and more aware that there are different ways of looking at life.

Summary

The therapeutic relationship is important in CBT, and it can certainly make the process of change much easier if you and your client have a strong and mutually respectful therapeutic bond. There are actions on the part of the therapist that may strengthen the therapeutic relationship that are also likely to have a beneficial impact on treatment outcome, such as taking care to check a client's understandings of the process of therapy (e.g. the need for an agenda, homework, completion of assessment tools, etc.), and to enhance the client's understanding of the rationale for certain tasks (Safran & Segal, 1996). As such, the therapist ought to take care to facilitate the therapeutic relationship, but in CBT we must maintain a balance so that the empirical nature of interventions and the action-oriented stance of CBT is not sacrificed too much in the early sessions. Often adopting an open and interested stance to how the client manages to live with their problems can successfully navigate therapy towards change and the development of a strong working alliance.

Learning Log: Reflection and Review
What have you gained from reading this chapter?

- What are your thoughts about the nature of the therapeutic relationship you develop with your clients? Do you engage in alliance-promoting behaviours and techniques in therapy? If so, list them for yourself and ask whether these are absolutely necessary in every case.
- Are there some clients that you have found difficult to like, and has this impacted upon your ability to help them? Can you think of what you could do differently and what you have learned from this experience?
- Think about the cohort attitudes of older people. Are there some additional actions you could take to understand more about the client group you will work with? Can you visit your local library and learn more about what life was like in your town before, during and after World War II? Could you watch popular movies from the 1940s to the 1960s when your clients were as young as you are now? Does Britain in the past look like a different country to you? How could you reflect on this and use it in your interactions with clients?

Further Reading

The following sources provide more in-depth coverage of topics raised in this chapter.

Safran, J. & Segal, Z. (1996). *Interpersonal process in cognitive therapy*. New Jersey: Jason Aronson.

For those wishing to understand more about cohort factors when working with older people, social history books may give additional insights.

Kynaston, D. (2007). *Austerity Britain (tales of a New Jerusalem) 1945–1951*. London: Bloomsbury.

Kynaston, D. (2013). *Modernity Britain (opening the box) 1957–1959*. London: Bloomsbury.

Marr, A. (2010). *The making of modern Britain*. London: MacMillan.

See also the BBC TV series *The making of modern Britain*.

Seven

Cognitive and Behavioural Interventions

Learning Objectives
By the end of this chapter you will:

- Understand the relationship between cognitions, emotions and behaviour in determining outcome of situations/experiences
- Understand how to identify and modify negative cognitions
- Use new age-friendly thought diaries to help people challenge cognitions
- Apply behavioural activation strategies with older people

Introduction

In CBT, cognitions are usually thoughts that can be stated in words that represent an individual's idiosyncratic thoughts, beliefs and interpretations/appraisals of stimuli. A lot of the therapeutic work in cognitive therapy sessions is devoted to the identification and modification of negative or dysfunctional thoughts. In cognitive restructuring, the client is taught self-monitoring skills to identify thoughts that are associated with negative mood and maladaptive behavioural responses. In emphasising cognitive restructuring, psychoeducation moves from discussing depression or anxiety towards a discussion of how thoughts, feelings and behaviour interact and how this is relevant to the client's current problem(s).

Automatic thoughts can be identified in a number of ways. During moments of strong emotion during therapy sessions the therapist can ask the client to state explicitly what thoughts went through their mind as their mood dropped. These thoughts are known as 'hot cognitions'.

You can help your client to identify negative thoughts by helping them to become more aware of changes (fluctuations) in their mood. When they notice that their emotion/mood has changed they can note down the (verbatim) thoughts that they are aware of. At first it may be sufficient just to get your client to record how often they feel upset, as being conscious of our thoughts and noting this down unedited (verbatim) is quite a challenging idea for clients to apprehend.

TABLE 7.1 *Typical thinking errors/distortions*

Cognitive distortion	Description of distortion	Example of distortion
Arbitrary inference (discounting the positive).	Drawing a specific conclusion in the absence of evidence or evidence to the contrary.	Client is visited in hospital by family and feels that she is a burden to them. 'They are only here out of duty.'
Selective abstraction (mental filter).	Focusing on a detail out of its context while ignoring more salient information.	Your client is given an appraisal at charity event that is extremely positive and yet ignores the praise and focuses on minor (constructive) criticisms.
Dichotomous reasoning (all or nothing thinking).	Propensity to categorise all experiences in one of two categories.	Client gets out of hospital and family doesn't visit immediately. They state that 'nobody cares for me, I am all alone in the world'.
Overgeneralisation.	Making more of the evidence than is warranted. Taking it to extremes.	Friend walking across the street fails to say hello. Client thinks, 'that's it, none of my friends want anything to do with me now'.
Personalisation	Propensity to relate external events to oneself.	Client finds out their oldest son has been arrested by police: 'I let my son down, I didn't act as a better role model. I'm a failure I didn't do my job as a dad properly.'
Magnification and minimisation.	Either exaggerating or downplaying the personal significance of an event for the client.	Minimisation: client conquers a phobia and states, 'its no big deal, most people aren't afraid of spiders'. Magnification: client forgets a friend's birthday and says 'I am a terrible, selfish person'.
Awfulising (catastrophising).	The propensity to think the worst possible outcomes for situations. Often the person ignores contradictory evidence, hence it is often linked with emotional reasoning.	Client has a headache and thinks, 'I am having a stroke, I'm going to die unless I get help'. Woman with a fear of elevators, is afraid that she will suffocate if an elevator is stuck, despite being 'trapped' in an elevator for 10 minutes in the past.
Emotional reasoning.	Person feels very anxious and apprehensive and assumes this means certain fears are about to be realised.	Goes to the shops and feels anxious and appraises the feelings as indicating that something terrible *is* happening: 'if I am feeling as bad as this at the shops, it must mean deep down something is really wrong'.

Attentional Biases in Cognitions

Attentional biases in the processing of emotionally congruent information/stimuli are evident in affective disorders, although they are different for depression and anxiety disorders (Mogg & Bradley, 2005). In anxiety disorders there is an enhanced attentional bias for external threat-related cues, whereas in depression people may find it hard to disengage attention from negative stimuli when it is apprehended (Gotlib & Joormann, 2010), suggesting that treatment approaches in depression and anxiety may need to take account of these attentional biases. However, the processing of salient information remains important. 'According to cognitive theories of emotion, cognitive appraisals determine whether an emotion is experienced and, if it is, which emotion is experienced. Thus, cognition is the primary route through which emotions are regulated' (Gotlib & Joormann, 2010: 301).

When a person's mood is low there are changes evident in their cognitive content. Thoughts become negative, and depressed people will typically make the types of errors in their thinking displayed in Table 7.1.

In depression, thoughts also have the character of being overgeneralised and lacking in specific details (Kuyken, 2006). This means that when working with negative attributions about situations or experiences it is important to get as much detail as possible. It is often important not to take the first answer when asking about a situation.

It's in the Eye of the Beholder: Cognitive Distortions

Helping clients to see a connection between their cognitions and their mood can explain how a situation led to a specific outcome for the individual, and that can help the client see that their behaviour was conditional upon these connections. This can be intriguing for clients as it provides interesting insights into the nature of their

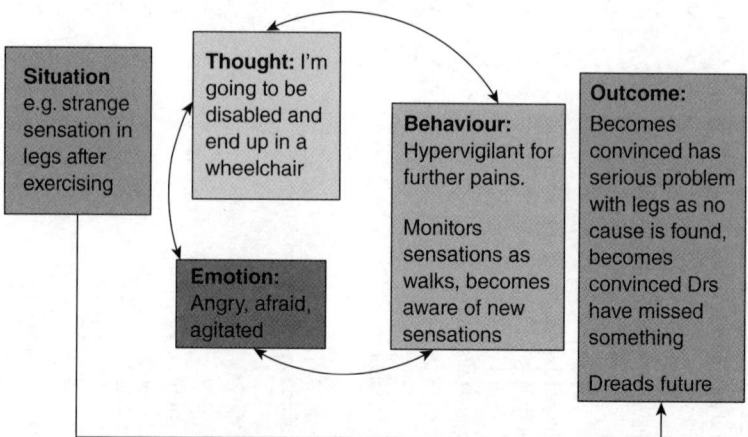

FIGURE 7.1 *Negative cognitive affective cycles*

problems. It is not the situation, but the meaning we attach to that situation/stimuli that determines its impact on our well-being. In Figure 7.1 we can see a situation in which a previously fit 81-year-old man notices uncomfortable sensations in his legs after exercising. After consulting his doctor and being sent for tests he convinced himself he has a serious degenerating illness.

The idiosyncratic nature of this connection can be understood by looking at the individual's thoughts, feelings and behaviours. The connection between situation and outcome is often the viewpoint clients bring into sessions. Clearly not everyone who develops uncomfortable sensations in their legs is convinced they will end up in a wheelchair. How the client makes sense of these sensations predicts their negative emotional response.

> Epictetus famously said: 'People are not disturbed by things, but by the view they take of them,' and 'It's not what happens to you, but how you react to it that matters.'

However, as the client is aged 81 and has an internalised negative stereotypical belief about ageing, this suggests he expects ageing to be about decrepitude and loss of function, and this may also explain the level of negative affect generated here.

Understanding the idiosyncratic personal meaning of events is a key task in figuring out how to help our clients. In CBT it is recognised that it is not the event per se that causes people problems, but their habitual way of making sense of things. The way people make sense of things may be determined by pre-existing vulnerabilities such as rigid and inflexible core beliefs or by a person's mood state, or in many cases both. We can help our clients by bringing two simple understandings to their attention.

1. A person's problems are caused more by the way they think about things, or the meanings attached to the event, rather than the event itself (see Figure 7.1).
2. Thoughts are not facts. No matter how much we believe something to be true this does not make it a fact.

Identifying and Challenging Cognitions

In CBT, examples of troubling cognitions might be 'I am a hypocrite' or 'I don't matter to anyone' or 'I have made such a struggle out of my life, yet other people happen to be getting on fine.' Usually when listening to an individual's cognitions, this can give an insight into the nature of their difficulties. It also offers a means of assessing the impact of these thoughts, beliefs and appraisals upon the individual. Thus, if a client has a negative cognition one would ordinarily expect them to experience a negative emotion. This assumption is one of the most basic elements of the Beck model of psychopathology in cognitive therapy.

Once the therapist has assessed cognitions in their most verbatim form possible (ask the client to tell you what exactly they thought in the situation) then it is important

A: Situation Describe the events that led to your unpleasant feelings: Where were you, what were you doing, who else was there?	B: Beliefs As your mood changed what thought was in your mind?	C: Emotions What are you feeling? (sad, angry, anxious, etc). How bad do you feel? 0–100% good?	D: Adaptive Thoughts What is a more helpful way to think about this situation?	E: Outcomes Re-rate the strength of the negative beliefs and feelings now
In choir practice, struggling to reach high notes.	I'm losing my singing voice 100%	Hopeless, devastated 100%	Not enjoying prog./others aren't enjoying it either. Prog of music is not suited to my voice, because voice is not trained. Choirmaster doesn't do a warm up for such a complex piece. Choirmaster's methods don't suit me.	Maybe not losing voice after all. If believed thought would have given up choir. If go with alternatives will continue to go to choir and make the best of the situation. Don't beat yourself up.

FIGURE 7.2   A typical DTR

to assess the consequent impact on the client's emotional state. This strategy in CBT is called *cognitive restructuring*. This means the therapist must ask clients to identify problematic appraisals of situations from their unique (idiosyncratic) point of view.

For example, Jean (78 years old) is afraid that the fuzzy sensations in her head mean she has a tumour. This fear is something that causes her distress. She is currently an inpatient in a psychiatric ward as her mood has been so low it was felt she may harm herself. When she tells the nurses on the ward that she is afraid she has a tumour the staff tend to reassure her, and while this works at the time, the fear persists. Jean has been meeting with a CBT therapist on a weekly basis while an inpatient. She describes her sensations and asks the therapist if they think she has a tumour. The therapist, using CBT techniques, asked Jean if she has ever known anyone with a brain tumour – she replied, her mother. Jean then de-escalated her own fears, as she was able to challenge her own thoughts about a tumour. In the following week Jean did not experience any further problems with this fear. This example tells us how powerful our thoughts can be and that clients don't need someone else to give them answers – sometimes it is about encouraging people to access their own existing wealth of knowledge.

Cognitive Restructuring

Cognitive restructuring is usually achieved through the use of thought diaries. Thought diaries have a wealth of names such as dysfunctional thought records (DTR) and unhelpful thought diary (UTD). The diaries take a range of forms, but usually have a similar format to Figure 7.2.

In the diary in Figure 7.2 a client has a fear that her voice is failing, and she attributes this as being largely due to her age. She tearfully related to her therapist that as she had lost her voice she could no longer continue singing in her choir. The therapist used standard techniques of asking about the evidence for this thought and evidence against it, to help the client assess how to make sense of the situation. The therapist did not take the stance of disputing what the client said, but merely adopted a collaborative curiosity in exploring this distressing situation with the client.

Clients more skilled at completing DTR are more likely to benefit from treatment for depression as the links between mood and cognition are clear, and those more skilled at capturing and challenging negative automatic thoughts may be better protected from relapse.

What Are You Asking Your Client to Do when Completing a DTR?

What you are expecting the client to do may seem to them like a very strange request. In effect you are asking them to think about thoughts, and writing these down in a DTR can be a challenging idea to many people, especially those who are depressed, as their confidence at mastering a new skill is likely to be low. This is

(Continued)

(Continued)

a complex idea, and therapists need to remember that as psychologists we may be used to the idea of reflection on ideas and thoughts – we might see this as a pleasant activity, but this may not appeal so easily to your client. It may need to be shaped up.

Introduce DTRs Using Successive Steps

As challenging thoughts and using DTRs are complex skills to master, it can be helpful to simplify the process as much as possible. If a weekly activity schedule (see Figure 7.3) has been used in early sessions, these can be useful for identifying negative thoughts especially if the therapist has asked the client to rate their activities for enjoyment or pleasure.

It is not unusual that different activities at different times provide different enjoyment ratings and these can be examined for thoughts about these activities on a weekly activity schedule (WAS). The enjoyment ratings for activities can be used within session to infer and discuss what sorts of thoughts were associated with the activity and what was it about these activities that merited their ratings.

Once the connections between thoughts and feelings are made, the introduction of a simple three-column DTR can be very useful, with columns allowing descriptions of situations, thoughts and feelings. Again, this technique should be practiced within the session using an example identified from the WAS that the client has completed as homework. Get the client to do as much work as possible on this themselves, but go slowly. It is important that you act as a coach here, giving the client frequent praise and encouragement, and acknowledging that it can be tough learning this new skill.

From these forms the therapist and client can graduate to using more complex forms, and the skill of cognitive restructuring can be more easily mastered. Thoughts being recorded in a DTR ought to have the following characteristics:

- They should be specific and focused. Often describing a discrete and identifiable situation that has provoked a strong emotional response.
- Emotions should be clearly identified with the event/situation and the associated thought.
- Thoughts ought to be written as close to verbatim as possible (in practice the therapist may capture a negative thought by the patient in session and model the completion of a diary by writing their verbatim thoughts in the appropriate column in the DTR).
- Responses or challenges to the negative automatic thought should be specific and linked to the negative thought. They ought to reflect a more compassionate or helpful response. The response should result in a reduction in negative affect.

Guided discovery can be useful when helping people identify and challenge negative automatic thoughts. Guided discovery is a process of having a client mentally 'retrace their steps' when recalling an event that elicited strong emotions. All the aspects of the

Weekly Activity Schedule.

	Mon .../.../...	Tues .../.../...	Wed .../.../...	Thurs .../.../...	Fri .../.../...	Sat .../.../...	Sun .../.../...
7 am – 8 am							
8 am – 9 am							
9 am – 10 am							
10 am – 11 am							
11 am – 12 pm							
12 pm – 1 pm							
1 pm – 2 pm							
2 pm – 3 pm							
3 pm – 4 pm							
4 pm – 5 pm							
5 pm – 7 pm							
7 pm onwards							

FIGURE 7.3   *Blank weekly activity schedule (WAS)*

Notes: Simply write down what you do in the times marked each day. One or two words are enough to describe what you do. For example, if you were doing housework at 10am–11am on Monday morning you would only need to write housework in the space provided. Please remember to bring this sheet with you at your next appointment. Your next appointment is scheduled for...../....../.....at......am/pm.

A copy of this figure is available to download from https://study.sagepub.com/laidlaw

distressing situation are recalled in order for the patient to access thoughts or images they experienced prior to a change in their emotional state.

The therapist can encourage the client to tell them where the person was when they felt sad, who else was there, and what was happening just at the moment their mood changed. It can be helpful to ask the client to try and picture themselves back in the situation, 'in your mind's eye'. At that point, it will be important to ask: 'can you see yourself back in the moment?' Once the client is able to affirm this, it may be useful to ask: 'when your mood changed, what thought went through your mind?', or 'when your mood changed, what did you say to yourself in your head?'

The therapist can model the completion of a diary form by writing parts of the diary in the relevant sections (situation, thoughts, feelings, etc.) in front of the client and then discussing the usefulness of this technique. Guided discovery is often discussed in connection with a procedure known as *Socratic questioning.*

Socratic questioning usually involves asking a client a series of open-ended questions that facilitate understanding and reveal maladaptive thought patterns. Padesky (1993) defined Socratic questioning as a method of questioning that: (i) involves asking clients questions that they have the knowledge to answer; (ii) brings clients' attention to information relevant to the topic being discussed, but which they were not accessing; (iii) involves moving clients from discussion of concrete issues to abstract issues and back again; in order that (iv) clients identify and apply new information such that they change previous conclusions or reconstruct ideas or beliefs.

Using Single-Event DTRs to Challenge Thoughts

Figure 7.4 illustrates a *new single-event* DTR. This type of DTR can be used either as the main format for thought challenging, or as an interim step to using a full five-column DTR as seen in Figure 7.2. In this incomplete DTR, Jennifer has recently had an operation on her knee. The operation itself was a great success and her surgeons are very positive that her mobility will improve as she recovers from the operation. When is she discharged, Jennifer's sense of hope quickly turns to despair as she feels neglected and alone. She brings this diary into her session with you.

When the therapist and client looked at the diary, Jennifer was encouraged to consider what evidence she could use to challenge her negative thoughts. Readers may wish to

Situation: Recovering from operation at home. No one has called me in ages!
Negative Thought: I'm a burden and I don't matter (to my daughters). I'm the bottom of the heap.
How does the negative thought make you feel? (tick as many as apply and rate intensity of feeling) Sad **x**   Angry **x**   Anxious   Ashamed **x** Guilty   Hopeless **x**   Other (write it here) **selfish**

Evidence for this thought	Evidence against this thought

Conclusion (What is a caring and helpful thing to say to yourself?):
Once you have reached your conclusion have your feelings changed? You are just wasting your time with me!   100% Has your intensity of feeling changed? Check on the scale here: 0%
Questions to help you examine your thoughts and feelings: First answer this question for yourself: Are you good, *or bad,* at predicting the future when you are upset? Now ask yourself. • If your negative thoughts were 100% true what would you *need* to do? • Are your thoughts always right? Could you be mistaken? • Is this the only way to think of this situation? • How does it help you to think this way? What's the effect of thinking this way? • Are there alternative ways to think about this? • What advice would you give a very good friend who thought this way? • Have you been in similar situations before and how did they turn out?

FIGURE 7.4   *Single-event DTR form*

A blank copy of this figure is available to download from https://study.sagepub.com/laidlaw

What evidence can I draw upon? Therapist DTR worksheet
Ways to address these (✓) ⊙ ☐   Historical data Has client felt like this before and how did that turn out? ⊙ ☐   Self-report (Thoughts aren't facts) Remind your client that even though we may believe our thoughts 100% this does not make them facts. Look for evidence that contradicts beliefs. ⊙ ☐   Behavioural Indices Ask the client if they have been passive or active. If passive remind them they can either continue to wait and feel more low, or are there actions they can take themselves? ⊙ ☐   Factual Data Ask the client for objective measurable data, that may be relevant to answering/challenging negative automatic thoughts ⊙ ☐   Psychoeducation Remind your client that when people feel low or anxious, mood congruent thoughts will be easier to bring to mind. Hence, when we are low we generate more thoughts about sad events, or previous slights, previous hurts etc. This can enflame our distress but rarely brings one close to constructive actions/resolutions. ⊙ ☐   Other There are many behavioural and cognitive options when dealing with negative thoughts. Perhaps you can suggest a homework task to explore understanding further (e.g. polling, *in-vivo* experiments, graded exposure etc.)
Options to challenge additional negative self-statements
Ways to address these (✓) ⊙ ☐   Cognitive restructuring ⊙ ☐   Direct self to give assurance and be more self accepting and compassionate ⊙ ☐   Behaviour experiment(s)/activation ⊙ ☐   Historical test of beliefs. (i.e client takes a belief and looks at evidence for and against this belief over their lifespan by evaluating its utility over different periods of the client's life. This activity should promote a compassionate acceptance of self. ⊙ ☐   other

FIGURE 7.5   *DTR worksheet*

A copy of this figure is available to download from https://study.sagepub.com/laidlaw

use the worksheet in Figure 7.5 to consider what evidence you could use to help Jennifer challenge her negative attribution that she is selfish and is wasting your time by taking up your sessions. The DTR worksheet in Figure 7.5 may be useful to you when working with incomplete DTRs and deciding how to approach the completion of these tasks.

As it turned out, following this session her eldest daughter visited, disconfirming her thoughts of being abandoned and uncared for. She felt quite ashamed for doubting her children's care, as they had been in touch before and after her hospitalisation. The hospital was a long distance from where her daughters live, and as they had family responsibilities it was impractical for them to visit, although they kept in touch by phone. When asked to say something compassionate towards herself in this situation, Jennifer responded:

'Its quite understandable. You had a rough childhood and felt neglected, so it immediately crops up that "its happening again" with the girls but it's the wrong context.'

In this instance, Jennifer was able to de-escalate the problem by herself. (It's often the case that people are able to do this, and as therapists we sometimes need to work harder at not jumping in too quickly with a ready-made solution.) She was able to see that because of her past experience she was primed to expect that her needs would be neglected. She knew that this was an old belief that she didn't need to accept any more.

Age-Related Negative Cognitions

In cognitive theory of CBT, the selective processing hypothesis (Clark et al., 1999), posits a *negativity bias* where individuals have a tendency to overlook positive information and selectively attend to negative stimuli. When people are depressed or anxious, negative expectations can develop into a dread about growing older (Laidlaw & Pachana, 2009). Therefore, when older people attribute their problems to ageing, this may reflect the operation of faulty information processing rather than factual appraisals of the reality of situations (Gotlib et al., 2004). While an older client may state with a compelling degree of conviction that ageing is the root cause of their problems, this is inconsistent with the norm for older people. Contrary to expectations, older people often express a high degree of life satisfaction.

Therapists are advised to become attuned to *age-related negative cognitions*, that is cognitions biased towards a negative appraisal of ageing congruent with pre-existing schemas reflecting negative stereotypes of ageing (see Figure 7.6). Examples of age-related negative cognitions are: 'all my problems are to do with being old', 'old age is a depressing time of life', 'at my age it is too late to change'. These types of cognitions can seem very realistic to therapists but are as amenable to change as any other negative automatic thought.

Negative Age Stereotypes As a Focus of Cognitive Intervention in CBT

Levy (2003; 2009) suggests that ageist societal attitudes internalised from a very young age and reinforced throughout adulthood become internalised negative age stereotypes (INSAs) reinforced by an attentional bias towards congruent negative information about ageing. These stereotypes become *self*-stereotypes. Levy (2009: 334) suggests that negative self-stereotypes become more salient for the individual as they encounter multiple alarming cues that act to endorse a view of themselves as 'old':

> The process of age stereotypes becoming self-relevant for individuals is facilitated by their encounters with a plethora of social cues, usually pejorative, that indicate they are old ... Unlike those who have been stigmatised since birth and consequently may acquire coping strategies from their subgroup, individuals tend to enter old age unprepared to resist negative age stereotypes.

These stereotypes act in similar ways to schemata in CBT, in that they are latent, maladaptive and rigidly held (Laidlaw, 2013a). Levy (2009) proposes that the utilisation of multiple pathways (affective, cognitive, behavioural and physical) is necessary for stereotype embodiment in individuals. Levy (2008) notes that older people endorsing negative age stereotypes report more negative age perceptions of self over time.

In a process akin to cognitive dissonance (Bohner & Dickel, 2011), an individual who attributes the nature and cause of their problems to ageing, rather than as symptoms of depression or anxiety, will be more inclined to seek out information congruent with this belief and deselect or avoid information that contradicts it. Levy (2008) offers partial support for this idea, providing evidence that older people with more 'rigid' personalities are more prone to adopt negative self-appraisals of ageing mediated by a negative age stereotypes. In further support Levy and Leifheit-Limson (2009) found a stereotype matching effect with the impact being greater when the content of stereotypes matched outcomes. Participants exposed to positive rather than negative age-stereotypes performed better on cognitive and physical stimuli.

By selectively attending to negative indicators of ageing, such as unwanted changes in physical appearance and loss of vitality, these are attributed to age rather than depression, and serve to activate the internalised negative age stereotype (the stress–diathesis is complete). A negative cycle develops as the individual becomes hyper-vigilant to other indicators of negative experiences of ageing, and these reinforce the individual's belief that old age is a depressing, fearful and unpleasant stage of life

In other words, negative events are attributed to the ageing process and the idiosyncratic explanatory construct reinforces an individual's negative appraisals so that older people attribute their problems to ageing rather than to any other cause. Older people then come to believe that their problems are unchangeable, as their *perceived problems associated with ageing become congruent with a negative age stereotype*. Self-stereotypes reflect the operation of a negativity bias (focused on ageing) in the thinking of older people.

A client with a range of problems and a reported low quality of life, which is communicated as 'ageing being a terrible stage', may reflect the operation of rigid and inflexible schemata (or negative self-stereotypes of ageing), and the impact of these beliefs could be underestimated in terms of their potential impact on therapy outcome. Clients themselves might not be fully aware of negative age stereotypes, accepting this as the norm. Congruent with the negative self-stereotype of ageing, an individual may misattribute symptoms of depression (sleep disturbance, anhedonia, hopelessness about the future, etc.) as being merely the negative consequences of ageing and may fail to seek help for a treatable illness.

Negative cognitions are more often age-related negative cognitions rather than more general negative cognitions (see Figure 7.6). The impact can be observed in terms of a simple A-B-C sequence that is standard within CBT, where the consequences for an individual (C) in this model are determined by the operation of a stress–diathesis (A–B). The stress–diathesis relationship is as follows: a client's pre-existing vulnerability to becoming distressed is their internalised negative age stereotype; if an activating event (stressor) is experienced that appears to reinforce a negative attribution to ageing, affective, behavioural and cognitive consequences will ensue (see Figures 7.6 and 7.7).

Negative events, such as changes to one's physical status or other relatively benign consequences of ageing, are seen as harbingers of more serious and irreversible negative aspects of growing older. As the individual attributes all negative events to ageing, a sense of hopelessness develops. In time a vicious cycle is set up where an individual expects negative consequences of ageing, which in turn explains poor quality of life as something to be endured rather than as poor quality of life being due to symptoms of depression. This can be communicated to the therapist as a plausible and coherent explanation of difficult life circumstances. This may in turn translate into hopelessness about change within the therapist.

The therapist and client collaboratively collect data relating to the development of negative affect from recent events in order to explore the operation of the INSA, and an explanatory theme of erroneous attribution of problems due to age may emerge. The operation of an age-related negative cycle is illustrated schematically in Figure 7.6.

A useful psychoeducational exercise at this point is to educate people about the impact of depression on cognitions and emotions, and the impact these may have on a person's confidence about their own personal agency and consequent confidence about the future (Bodner, 2009). The therapist should note that using demographic change to educate depressed and anxious older people is *not recommended*, as it tends to either make people feel inadequate as it appears most people are managing to age more effectively than they are, or it makes people more anxious as they assume they have more years of misery ahead of them.

Cognitive restructuring is useful here, and beliefs are more likely to change if a client is helped to examine evidence from a perspective other than their own. In other words, ask your client to apply their negative age attributions to a very good friend in distress, and examine this approach for its utility.

Because it is hypothesised that the INSA operates much like a core belief, it is recommended therapists use standard techniques for schema change, such as a historical test of beliefs, continuum theory, seeing core beliefs as self-prejudice to test the reality

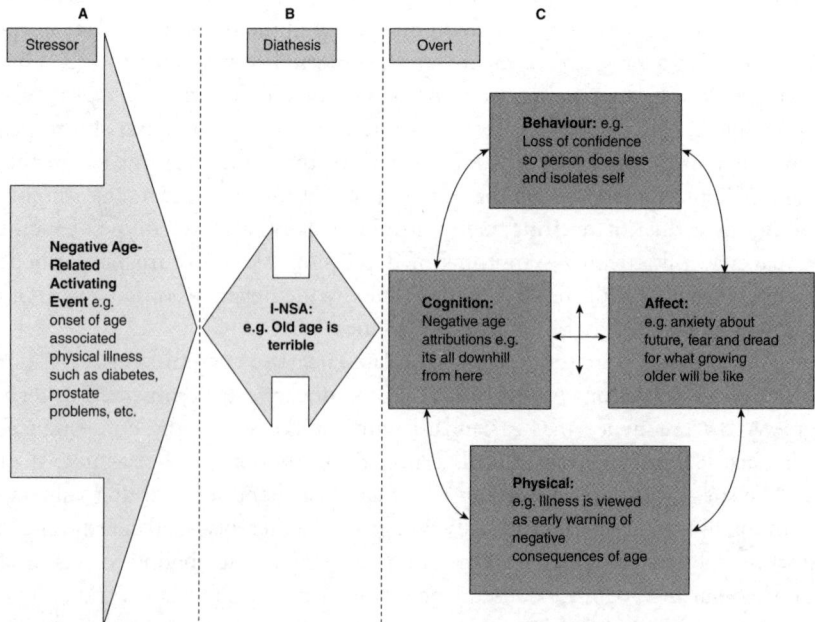

FIGURE 7.6 *Vicious cycle of age-related cognitive process errors activated by age-related negative event*

A blank copy of this figure is available to download from https://study.sagepub.com/laidlaw

of the INSA. Treating the INSA as a core belief allows the therapist to engage the client in an exploration of the evidence for this belief and to identify a possible more helpful belief about ageing (e.g. 'ageing isn't always easy, but its not all bad').

As an example of an INSA complicating treatment for depression, Mrs Gray is depressed and convinced her life is over and there is nothing to look forward to, as the future she envisages is filled with decline and further loss. She is convinced that she is irrelevant to significant others (see case example below). As she says this with 100 per cent certainty, it seems disrespectful and unempathic for the therapist to dispute Mrs Gray's distressing experience. Nevertheless, a negative cognitive triad (Beck et al., 1979) is evident in her narrative:

- Self – old and decrepit
- Future – filled with loss and decline
- Others – nobody cares for me and about me

A sensitive empathic clinician may engage this client in an exploration of the impact of her processing of information (see Table 7.2 for a summary of cognitive and behavioural intervention).

Case Example: Age-Related Negative Cognitions

Mrs Gray is 82 years old, and she was widowed two years ago when her husband, whom she had cared for, died quite suddenly. Although she was her husband's primary carer, she has mobility problems as she has arthritis and walks with the aid of two sticks. She has been feeling quite low lately, saying that 'nobody needs me' and that if she passed from this world to the next it would not trouble anyone. She is also the last of her cohort of friends, who have all died. 'I'm the only one of my generation … It is upsetting. I'm the next to go.' All of what Mrs Gray says is factually correct. It is true

TABLE 7.2 *Summary of interventions with Mrs Gray's age-related cognition*

Thought:
I am redundant [not needed] and would pass from this world without troubling anyone.
Cognitive strategies:
Thoughts aren't facts. Even though it feels like it is 100 per cent true this does not mean it would be true. So when you die do you expect your family to be 'untroubled'?
How does thinking this way help you? What impact does it have on your mood and on your motivations to do things?
Before you were depressed, how might you have thought about this?
What is the evidence for (and against) the idea you are redundant?
Is there an alternative way to think about it?
If this was a very dear friend who said this about themselves, how would you reply?
Behavioural strategies:
Gain more information about client perception of events (e.g. do polling – ask a family member if they think person is not needed by the family anymore).
Measure how much client can actually do (e.g. set up a behavioural experiment to see what obstacles are actually 'insurmountable').

that as the last of cohort of friends born in the same era and she will be the next to go, but no one has a crystal ball for the future. It is easy to become convinced that the negative appraisal of the situation by Mrs Gray is both accurate and understandable. However, therapists ought to remind themselves that when a person is depressed their view of the current situation and the future is coloured by negativity (see Figure 7.7).

Thoughts can seem very plausible when expressed by depressed people. When Mrs Gray says 'They'd get by perfectly well without me. This is the way I feel. There's no point being here,' the truth is that she is conjecturing an opinion of what her daughters will think and feel. Moreover, just because she says there is no point in her being here doesn't mean that there is no point. Importantly, the impact of these thoughts is power-fully negative, and unless addressed will maintain her low mood. They could easily be tested, and this can be done as a homework task. The therapist may wish to discuss with their clients how they can obtain a factual description of the situation (in this case, the client spoke with her daughters and corrected her erroneous assumptions).

Mrs Gray has two daughters, both of whom she is close to. One daughter in particular appears to need her mother for support. Thus, asking what Mrs Gray means when she says 'nobody needs me' is a good starting point. In this case Mrs Gray has a narrow view of being needed from when she was the mother providing for her family. Mrs Gray needs to update her model of how she can remain needed in a different but equally important way. She was encouraged to talk to her daugh-ters about her sense of redundancy. Her daughters were very clear that she was still needed by them. As one of her daughters was going through a divorce, she was being relied upon for moral support and on occasion for childcare support. With careful exploration of evidence for and against her belief that she was not needed, Mrs Gray was able to see that at the very least her daughter would miss her, stat-ing that 'Margaret needs me just now. I'm the only one she chats things over with. She'd miss me.'

Mrs Gray was also encouraged to develop a behavioural schedule to increase pleasurable activities, and over the course of three months her BDI score dropped from 32 to 20. As she increased her activity levels she became more confident, and noted that the more she did the more she felt like doing. Her BDI score reduced further to 13. She no longer felt redundant and started enjoying life again, pushing the boundaries of what she could do. On reflection, Mrs Gray was able to state: 'I can do more than I perhaps thought I could.'

Thus, even people with 'real' problems who have physical health challenges and are among the oldest-old can still challenge their thoughts. It is also important for therapists to be aware that even when there seems to be a 'factual basis' for the negative mood state, there is always room for improvement when negative cognitions are present.

Remember that even when a person believes their thoughts 100 per cent, and no matter how compelling or how consistent the story seems, people are reporting their perceptions of the facts and the products of their thoughts.

No matter how convincing a person's report is, thoughts are not facts (Overholser, 1995). Always keep an open mind for the possibility of change.

Mrs Gray's case is a good example of a person's pre-existing internalised stereotype of ageing acting as a diathesis (pre-existing vulnerability) activated by negative events attributed to ageing. This perception leads an individual to become convinced that their problems are not symptoms of depression or anxiety but are negative consequence of ageing. This process is illustrated in Figure 7.7 (note that the physical component here is dispensed with as the physical elements are contained within the activating event itself).

Remember, a depressed person's attribution about the future is likely to reflect information processing errors (the negativity bias) rather than a realistic evaluation (Gotlib et al., 2004). Depressed individuals have a specific pattern of selective biased processing of emotional stimuli, which intensifies attention to negative stimuli and the inability to disengage from negative stimuli resulting in emotion dysregulation (Gotlib & Joormann, 2010). Imagine how you would treat thoughts about the future as voiced by a 32 year old rather than an 82 year old, and proceed accordingly.

Behavioural Activation in CBT

Behavioural approaches are integral to CBT. Currently researchers (Lejuez et al., 2001; Martell et al., 2010) stress the use of behavioural activation (BA) as a treatment for depression in its own right. While there is a lot of merit in this approach, CBT therapists are reliant upon active behavioural interventions for optimal treatment outcome (see the example of Mrs Cameron in Chapter 10).

'BA is based on the premise that problems in vulnerable individuals' lives reduce their ability to experience reward from their environments, leading to the symptoms

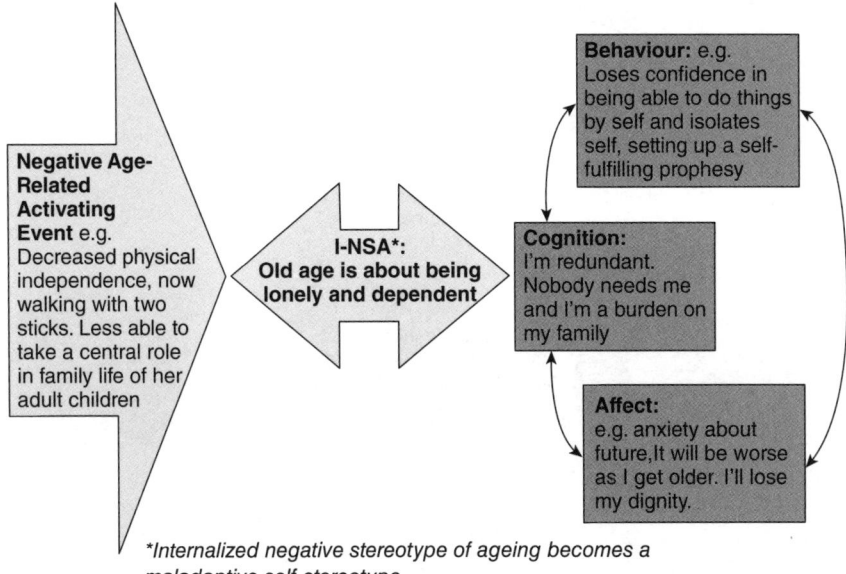

Internalized negative stereotype of ageing becomes a maladaptive self-stereotype

FIGURE 7.7   *Mrs Gray's vicious cycle of age-related cognitions*

and behaviors that we classify as depression' (Martell et al., 2010: 21). This provides an important behavioural principle: problems are located within the environment and in how the individual engages with the environment. The environment in behavioural terms means both the internal environment (how the person feels, stress levels, etc.) and the external environment (understimulating or overstimulating). Individuals can moderate their internal environment (e.g. by examining and challenging their attributions) but cannot necessarily moderate the external environment (although they can change the way they respond to or approach stressors in the environment). Thus, when using behavioural approaches in CBT one needs to be mindful of the individual's idiosyncratic meaning attached to events – cognitive elements are just as essential as behavioural elements for outcome in CBT.

As a person's mood level drops, a vicious cycle develops (see Figure 7.8) that reduces the availability of positive reinforcers for the client (Lewinsohn et al., 1986). Initially, carers, relatives, friends, etc., are usually sympathetic and give the person a lot of empathy. However, this rarely resolves problems (Lejuez et al., 2001) and the person's low mood can become increasingly aversive to others, and as such the client tends to become more isolated further reducing mood (see Figure 7.8).

Introducing the depression spiral is useful in a number of ways: first, it highlights the important role behaviour may play in the development of depression, and sets up

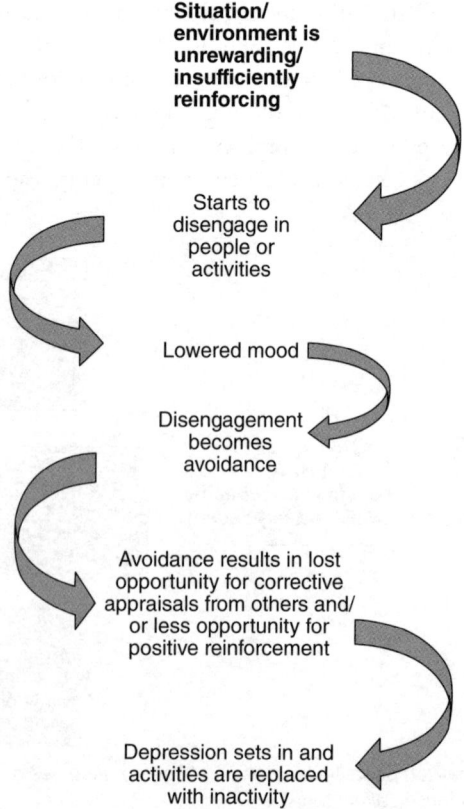

Situation/environment is unrewarding/insufficiently reinforcing

Starts to disengage in people or activities

Lowered mood

Disengagement becomes avoidance

Avoidance results in lost opportunity for corrective appraisals from others and/or less opportunity for positive reinforcement

Depression sets in and activities are replaced with inactivity

FIGURE 7.8 *The depression spiral*

a rationale for introducing BA or pleasant events scheduling (PES) as a treatment intervention; second, it is non-judgemental and non-blaming; third, as the client's understanding of depression sets in gradually, recovery means reversing the spiral and must therefore also occur gradually so that realistic goals and timescales are understood by the client. Reversing the depression spiral is not easy, as clients will have cut back on activities and hobbies and cut themselves off from friends who may provide positive affirmation (Lewinsohn et al., 1986; Lejuez et al., 2011; Martell et al., 2010).

> When using BA in CBT it is important to establish an accurate baseline for activity before setting a new goal for your client. It is important to build in success by starting small and going slow. Remember, your client will have a lot of past 'failures' at trying to get themselves motivated, and many of these will be due to an overambitious goal for progress. If the client can make big changes without coming to therapy they don't need your help!

People who are depressed are unlikely to be enthusiastic about an approach that requires them to engage in action, as they fear their actions will result in failure and this expectation fuels avoidance behaviour. Alternatively, clients set expectations for change so high that they reinforce a sense of failure. For example, Mr Weiss was a 69-year-old businessman with a number of small stores. He was referred because he was depressed and spent most mornings in bed. He also experienced insomnia, so many of his hours in bed were spent ruminating about himself and his inability to 'fix' himself. When the therapist suggested he reduce these depression-inducing behaviours he agreed to try, but was not optimistic that this approach would help as it seemed so simplistic. Mr Weiss was keen to make a plan to get out of bed at 9.00 a.m. the next morning in order that he could 'get my life back on track'. The therapist asked the client how often he had risen at 9.00 a.m. in the past three weeks. Mr Weiss stated that he had not been out of bed before midday for many weeks. The therapist carefully gained accurate information about the hour Mr Weiss typically got out of bed and made a plan with him to attempt to rise fifteen minutes earlier, on at least three occasions over the following week. While Mr Weiss was unhappy at the low goal set for him, his therapist reminded him that this task was a behavioural experiment to understand more about the impact of depression. Importantly, the therapist reminded the client that if he was able to rise from bed by 9.00 a.m. every morning he would already be doing that, and would not need to be attending appointments. The therapist joins the client's team as his coach, not as an expert telling him what to do. This is an important principle (Martell et al., 2010), as it also means that any success is due to the hard work of the client, not the expertise of the therapist.

The key strategy in BA is that frequency and occurrence of pleasant events are increased. Graded exposure and graded hierarchies are necessary tools to help a client get started on activities, and problem solving is also necessary in order to overcome practical obstacles to the client engaging in tasks. Socratic exploration of what the client can gain by engaging in behavioural experiments facilitates client self-reinforcement regarding progress made (see also Chapter 7).

BA is described in detail in both Martell et al. (2010) and Lejuez et al. (2011), who describe a briefer version of BA called Behavioural Activation for Depression (BATD).

A very useful tool in BA is a WAS. As a first step you can ask your client to complete a WAS as a homework task in order to create a baseline of your client's current activity level. A snapshot of a WAS is illustrated in Figure 7.9.

Time	Mon	Tues	Wed	Thurs	Fri	Sat	Sun
8.00	read paper	read paper	Papers	Read paper	Stayed in bed	Stayed in bed	Stayed in bed
9.00	housework	housework	walked dog	Walked to newsagent	in bed	Stayed in bed	Stayed in bed
10.00	watched tv	watched tv	shopping	Watched tv	In bed	Stayed in bed	Stayed in bed
11.00	read paper	read paper	Grandkids visit	Talked on phone	In bed	Stayed in bed	Stayed in bed
12.00	lunch	lunch	childminding Grandkids	childminding Grandkids	In bed	read paper	read paper
1.00	Exercise bike	Exercise bike	watched tv	childminding Grandkids	Fixed lunch	Exercise bike	read paper
2.00	watched tv	watched tv	knitted	Watched tv	Watched tv	Watched tv	Went for walk

FIGURE 7.9   *Snapshot of a WAS as a measure of activity levels*

The WAS gives you an idea of the person's activity. Importantly, it gives you a measure of how much or how little they are doing. A WAS gives insights into your client's routine, providing useful information about disruption to appetite and sleep patterns. You can also use it in later sessions to get the person to record mastery and pleasure:

- Mastery is a sense of achievement gained from doing something
- Pleasure is an indication of enjoyment gained from doing something (Laidlaw et al., 2003)

In practice, it is usually more useful to ask your client to record pleasure ratings (from 0–10, with 0 being no enjoyment/pleasure at all and 10 being total enjoyment), and only use mastery if this is seen as an important indicator for the individual. When assessing the WAS with your client you may wish to ask them the following:

1. What was the best part (high point) of your week (from WAS)?
2. What was the worst part (low point) of the week?
3. Think about what made these your best and worst points. How could you change things?

From Figure 7.9 it should be noted that there is a very low rate of pleasant events and the client is quite passive and inactive. There is also a lack of variety in the week. These could be important targets when asking the client how they might like things to change, and what they would do differently if they weren't depressed. It can be illustrative for the therapist to ask the client if the current WAS is different from before they were depressed. It can be important to establish whether their depressed state is the norm for the client, and to develop a motivation to return to a more balanced way of living.

Identifying Pleasant Events in BA

It is important to help your client recognise the link between mood and activity level. Identifying potentially pleasant events means finding activities that people like to do, then encouraging people to do them so they feel better.

Pleasant events needn't be big events like going on holiday or buying an expensive gift for oneself. In fact, many people have small pleasant events that they take for granted, like reading a novel or having a leisurely lunch with friends. 'Pottering' about in the garden or washing the car can be pleasant events for many people.

> Anything that a person likes to do, and is rewarding for them, is a pleasant event.

Introducing a few extra pleasant events into a person's week can make a big difference to the quality of their lives and to the quality of their mood. It is much better to help the person focus on building up hobbies or behaviours they have stopped doing which they have not yet replaced with another activity. It is a good idea to start this as soon as possible.

Jennifer was referred for CBT as she was not responding to antidepressant medications and had stopped going to her local choir, dance class and painting group. In discussion with her therapist, Jennifer agreed to start increasing her activities by focusing on re-engaging with her choir, as this was the most meaningful activity for her. The choir activity was seasonal and had started in September. Jennifer had started seeing her therapist in early November. She had a choice: she could rejoin the choir before December, as the choir was preparing for the Christmas carol concert, or she could wait to rejoin the choir in January. Jennifer completed a pros and cons sheet with her therapist and decided to rejoin the choir straight away. The therapist problem-solved the implementation of this strategy with Jennifer in advance, and she successfully completed this task despite it being stressful. She said that 'It was lovely to see people again. People happy to see me back.' When her therapist asked what she gained by going back, she replied: 'It gives me joy. I love singing, I meet other people,' and it 'shows I made an effort, maybe I'm not so bad at all.'

Increasing Activity Can Be Challenging

> Remember, even activities that are enjoyable and meaningful for your client may also be stressful.

Items on a pleasant events list ought to be meaningful for the client, but pleasurable events may provoke stress as the client takes them up again after a break from doing them regularly.

Arthur was a keen painter, but as he took on the primary caregiver role for his wife as she developed dementia he stopped painting. After she died, the thought of painting again was very challenging as he thought he may not be able to paint as well as before. As a first step, Arthur was encouraged to just stretch some canvasses. Much later on he returned to painting, but through a successive series of steps. Near the end of treatment this is what he said about eventually going back to painting: 'I felt terrified, and it was difficult to get myself to do it. I thought, I'll never do it.' 'Doing it gives you a sense of confidence, I thought it had gone for good and it hasn't; it's back.'

Creating a List of Pleasant Events

In BA it is important to get the client to list things they most enjoy doing. Table 7.3 can be useful for this purpose.

TABLE 7.3   *BA list of pleasant events*

Top 5 list of pleasant events (activities) that I enjoy:	When did I last do these?
1.	
2.	
3.	
4.	
5.	

A copy of this table is available to download from https://study.sagepub.com/laidlaw

Tracking a Client's List of Pleasant Events

After having your client identify their top-five list, each day ask them to complete the WAS as before, but instead mark the occurrence of events from their top-five list using some indicator such as an asterisk. Alternatively, clients may prefer to complete a BA pleasant events tracking form (see Table 7.4). This form helps your client record how often they have engaged in pleasant activities and how enjoyable this has been. In the example below, the client currently gets less enjoyment watching golf on the TV. They castigate themselves for not doing something more active.

Arthur says: 'Watching the golf or whatever sport activity is an excuse to waste time. I'm just being lazy.' However, this is a pleasant activity for him and if he gives himself permission he may enjoy the sport, and it provides an interest for him to follow when a competition is on. His therapist asked what he might get out of watching TV. Arthur replied: 'Thrill in watching the players, degree of satisfaction in watching tournament unfold and following certain players, and gives you a rest from your worries. It's a switch-off.' Sometimes in BA the balance has to be struck in finding opportunities for the client to be more self-soothing and to be more compassionate towards themselves.

TABLE 7.4   *BA pleasant events tracking form*

Activities	Mon	Tues	Wed	Thurs	Fri	Sat	Sun	Enjoyment level 0–10
Washing the car	✓		✓		✓			7
Working in garden		✓		✓			✓	5
Going for a walk	✓	✓			✓	✓	✓	7
Watching golf on TV		✓	✓		✓			3
Daily total	2	3	2	1	3	1	2	

TABLE 7.5   *Homework/behaviour experiment pre-planning worksheet*

Preparation for homework activity	Internal obstacle This can be your thoughts, emotional response or physical response.	External obstacle This can be an aspect that is outside your control (e.g. you may need to ask people to do something in order that you can start your task).
Are there obstacles to starting my activity/task Are there obstacles to completing my activity/task When do I plan to do this task?		

Copies of these tables are available to download from https://study.sagepub.com/laidlaw

Identifying Obstacles to Engaging in Pleasant Events

It is not uncommon for clients to feel overwhelmed by starting BA or by starting to try to change their problems. It may be useful (using Socratic questioning) to identify how they might benefit from doing these activities. You may want to construct a pros and cons form to help them identify what they will gain from doing this. Table 7.5 is a pre-homework chart you may wish to use with clients before they leave your session.

Making the Connection Between Mood Level and PE

The final step in helping your client/patient to increase their activity levels is getting them to see that taking part in pleasant activities has a positive effect on their mood. The easiest and most efficient way of doing this is to combine the information you have from the WAS or from the pleasant events tracking form, and look at mood ratings from a standardised questionnaire such as the BDI/GDS or GAD-7/GAS.

Summary and Conclusions

Using cognitive and behavioural techniques in CBT is best understood as having two different but complementary tools that help you to help your client. Both elements of C and B are indivisible and indispensable in CBT. When working with clients at the start of therapy you may be more likely to use BA, but even here it is unlikely that you will be completely effective if you do not use cognitive restructuring and Socratic questioning. The reality is that CBT is not a talking cure but a 'doing cure'. Therefore, it requires you to be directive and problem-oriented. Both elements of CBT are necessary for you to meet your goals with your client.

Learning Log: Reflection and Review

- CBT works better if you understand the theory as well as the practice. Use some CPD time to become more familiar with the cognitive theory.
- Review self-help materials that you use for clients with depression and anxiety. Can you create some user-friendly versions of diaries and worksheets for use with your clients?
- Refresh your knowledge by going back over the classic CBT text by Beck et al. (1979). Notice how behavioural and cognitive elements are equally important.

Further Reading

The following sources provide more in-depth coverage of topics raised in this chapter.

Dryden, W. & Branch, R. (Eds.). (2012). *The CBT handbook*. London: SAGE.

Gallagher-Thompson, D., Steffen, A., & Thompson, L. W. (Eds.) (2008). *Handbook of behavioral and cognitive therapies with older adults*. New York: John Wiley & Sons.

Lewinsohn, P. M., Munoz, R. F., Youngren, M. A., & Zeiss, A. M. (1986). *Control your depression*. New York: Prentice Hall.

Martell, C. R., Dimidjian, S., & Herman-Dunn, R. (2010). *Behavioral activation for depression: a clinician's guide*. New York: Guilford Press.

Eight

Age-Appropriate CBT: Case Conceptualisation with Older People

Learning Objectives

By the end of this chapter you will:

- Understand the need for an age-appropriate case conceptualisation of CBT with older people unique to every client
- Appreciate what information you need to gather in order to develop a successful case conceptualisation
- Appreciate the need for different levels of case conceptualisation when working with older people

Introduction

A case conceptualisation is an individualised clinical theory that links overt symptoms presented at the time of a depression or anxiety episode with underlying, or covert, issues important to understanding the wider context of a client's difficulties. Case conceptualisations provide an explanatory context linking longstanding vulnerability to the development of problems within the persistent and recurrent nature of presenting problems across an individual's own lifespan. As such, a case conceptualisation is both descriptive and predictive. It describes how the person experiences the world and how they may be inclined to respond to stimuli in their environment through the operation of pre-existing and maladaptive belief structures (schemata). It can therefore predict difficulties and obstacles. It may be useful for the therapist to reflect on what aspects of therapy may be challenging for their client based upon the case conceptualisation. Thus, someone who holds a strong belief that they are a 'failure' are probably going to have a heightened tendency to avoid risk of failure to the extent that their cognitions and behaviours become self-defeating. An example of this is when clients fail to fully engage in therapy in case they fail. Evidence for this can be understood within a developmental perspective and patterns of behaviour can be pointed out to the client in sessions so they can be given responsibility to change. The therapist who conceptualises is likely to be able to anticipate challenges and to be able to work more collaboratively with the client, because they have actively sought to understand them. It also provides you with a way to deal with less typical presentations.

Case conceptualisation is now standard in any CBT textbook and is part of the range of competences identified by Roth and Pilling (2007) in their competence model. It is also a standard feature of any CBT treatment – see box on core principles of CBT.

Core Principles of CBT

1. Use of an *agenda* to structure your sessions
2. Primary use of *collaborative empiricism* to test ideas out
3. *Psychoeducation* is used at the start of treatment, and throughout as necessary, in order that the therapeutic alliance is based upon mutuality, respect and collaboration (the therapist acts as coach and not as expert)
4. The main way to explore your client's world view is the use of *Socratic questioning*
5. All treatment is based upon an individualised *cognitive case conceptualisation/formulation*
6. *Homework* is the primary means of generalising the benefits of treatment beyond individual sessions, and is agreed at the end of every session and reviewed at the start of the next

---

Even introductory texts on CBT don't reduce treatment down to a set of techniques and technologies. As anxiety and depression in later life often present together or are comorbid with other physical health conditions, there may not always be a simple conceptualisation framework that you can use with older people (Laidlaw et al., 2004). It can therefore sometimes be a challenge to individualise CBT treatment to meet the needs of older people, and at the same time practice therapy that adheres to the core principles of CBT and is consistent with evidence-based guidelines. In these challenging circumstances you may find yourself needing to translate theory into practice by working at the level of 'meta-competences' – that is, when 'Competent practitioners need to be able to implement higher-order links between theory and practice in order to plan and, where necessary, to adapt therapy to the needs of individual clients' (Roth & Pilling, 2007: 9).

A key skill to successfully navigate these potential difficulties is the ability to complete case conceptualisations. Case conceptualisations also ensure you stay 'cognitive' so you don't lose focus in planning psychologically helpful interventions that remain within the modality of the CBT interventions. Kuyken et al. (2009) note that case conceptualisations can help the therapist work collaboratively with clients with complex issues in three ways:

1. Describe presenting issues (overt symptoms and current problems)
2. Understand problems in ways that are cognitive and behavioural (thus focus on cognitive and behavioural strategies to reduce distress)
3. Develop a constructive focus to relieve distress and build on the client's pre-existing strengths and increase resilience (thus the focus is on empowering clients to recognise their positive attributes)

While there is little compelling evidence that case conceptualisation improves treatment outcomes, it is an important means of linking theory to practice and may therefore function to improve the extent to which therapists adhere to the evidence base (Kuyken et al., 2009). Case conceptualisation may also strengthen the therapeutic alliance, and it may be a useful tool in ensuring that therapists avoid therapeutic drift (Waller, 2009).

Therapeutic drift is when the therapist 'drifts' away from using standard procedures that adhere to the guiding principles of the main mode of therapy they profess to practice, thus reducing the likelihood that treatment will be successful (Waller, 2009). It may occur for a number of reasons, such as lack of adequate knowledge and skill in evidence-based approaches and because of a lack of supervision. To avoid falling into the traps of therapeutic drift you may wish to reflect on how many of the core principles of CBT you utilise in your sessions at a routine level. The routine use of a tool such as the Cognitive Therapy Rating Scale-Revised (Blackburn et al., 2001) is also a good thing to bring into your supervision sessions.

What are Case Conceptualisations?

Case conceptualisations are clinical theories that link error in cognitive content, processing errors and the operation of schemata linked to matching stressors within

CBT is Individually Tailored	A case conceptualization (CC) in CBT is a clinical theory about the individual that explains the nature of their problems, currently and historically and is predictive of potential challenges/obstacles towards optimal treatment progression. It is **bespoke** to the individual and is not pre-manufactured so the CC you share with your client should only describe the individual and their experiences.
	If possible the therapist should attempt to write a single sentence summarizing the nature of the client's current problems, their development and maintenance.

Prior to discussing your conceptualization with your client you may wish to organize your thoughts by asking yourself a few key questions:

1. Are there identifiable predispositions your client possesses that are important for understanding their current difficulties?
2. Are there identifiable precipitants that are important for the development and maintenance of the client's current problems?
3. Are there identifiable cognitions, beliefs and linked behaviours that explain the level of distress your client experiences currently?

FIGURE 8.1   *CBT is individually tailored*

the wider context of the internal and external environment affecting the individual. It is important that this is bespoke to the individual and is not generic and pre-manufactured (see Figure 8.1).

> Conceptualisation has a confusing set of different names meaning the same thing. In CBT, when developing a formulation, a conceptualisation or a case conceptualisation, you are essentially doing the same thing. At first this technique was called formulation, but increasingly the term case conceptualisation is used instead.

In CBT, case conceptualisation/formulation is a key skill and it may take a while before a therapist becomes comfortable with completing them. Nonetheless, it is essential to complete a conceptualisation as soon as possible (i.e. from the end of the third to fifth session onwards in the case of depression), otherwise your treatment is likely to be reactive rather than proactive. In other words, you are likely to remain in the dark about the motivations and vulnerabilities of your client.

Preparing for Conceptualisation

There is a range of information useful in any conceptualisation. The following are just an indication of the sorts of information that you may wish to draw upon:

- Diagnostic information may influence but not determine a conceptualisation.
- Early experiences/important events in adulthood. This extends well into adulthood and should not be confined to adolescence or early adulthood.
- Current stressors/current reasons for treatment/problem list.
- Themes arising from habitual negative thoughts.
- Habitual forms of information processing errors.
- Reflections on client style of relating both within the sessions and in relationships outside therapy.
- Coping strategies used to deal with current problem, and proactive ability to deal with crises over a lifetime.

You might wish to take a staged approach to gathering the information for your conceptualisation. Thus, by successive approximation you might:

1. Look at the problem list

   o Symptom lists
   o Overt versus covert difficulties
   o Timelines

2. Consider the content of automatic thoughts

   o Look for themes, e.g. weakness, failure

3. Prepare mini hypotheses/working hypotheses

   o 'I wonder if this makes sense to you . . .'

4. Propose homework tasks

   o Be creative, use personalised ideas

When conceptualising, it is usual to have a specific therapeutic model in mind. The Beck model of psychopathology (Beck et al., 1979) is perhaps the best-known model for CBT, and especially so for depression (see Figure 8.2). It is a stress–diathesis model, meaning that everyone has a particular vulnerability (the diathesis), or set of vulnerabilities, that may become activated in a stressful situation. An individual may not be aware of these vulnerabilities until they are activated by congruent stressors, and may react badly in specific situations that contribute to an individual's increased sense of alarm or distress.

The Beck model of psychopathology provides a comprehensive explanation of why certain situations or stressors provoke certain responses in some individuals but not in others. The model is often used as the basis for a basic case conceptualisation in therapy. It is a good fit for depression, but much less so for other conditions and with clinical populations other than adults of working age.

In using this model for a case conceptualisation, you need to be able to fill in any gaps in your knowledge about the client. This may be especially so with regard to covert beliefs at the start of treatment.

The Beck model is a dual layer model. The overt (symptom) level comprises the symptoms or the client's perception of the problem, and this is usually linked with a recent activating event. Schemata (covert) level comprises the beliefs, rules and assumptions your client holds about themselves, the world and others.

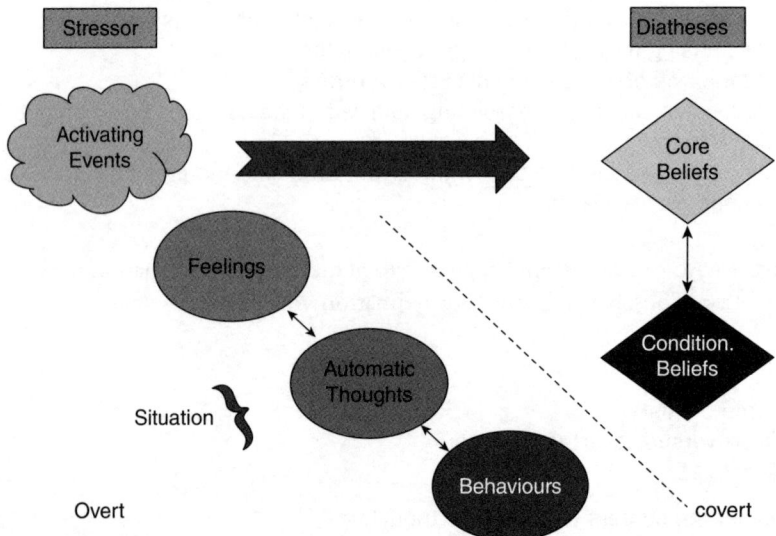

FIGURE 8.2 *Beck's model of psychopathology*

Step One

Thus, step one in conceptualisation is understanding reasons for the client presenting in your office with their problems. Ask yourself: why is the client needing help with this problem, why now?

Step Two

The second step is to understand the current symptoms of depression or anxiety in terms of thoughts, feelings and behaviour and how this may be linked with a pre-existing vulnerability such as a rigid maladaptive core belief. You may find it useful to complete the worksheet in Figure 8.3.

Step Three

The third step in conceptualisation is a little more complicated and requires you to process clinical information from a range of sources. This is where you think about the factors that 'underly' a person's presentation. It may also provide some important clues as to obstacles that can present in therapy in terms of more rigid beliefs.

Figure 8.4 provides a way to hypothesise about the more enduring nature of a client's difficulties. You can use this sheet to make sense of the types of cognition errors your client habitually makes, and it may provide you with a means of understanding your client's appraisal.

It may be helpful to try to summarise all this information on one single sheet – see the worksheet in Figure 8.5. This schematic contains all the elements of the model above but does so in a way that may help you organise your thoughts. It can be completed in stages and can also be used as a homework task for your client to complete.

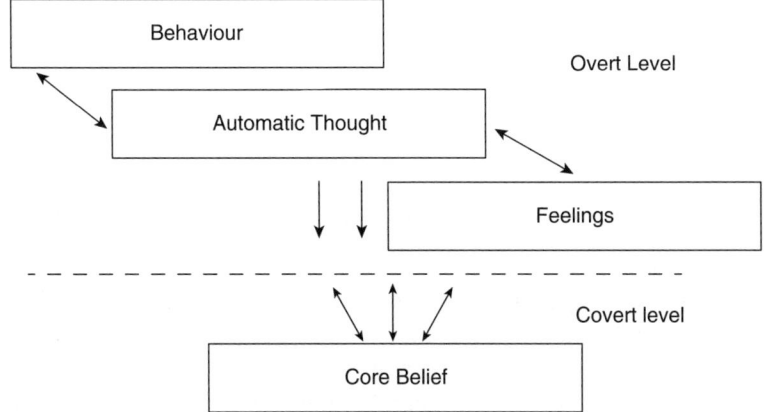

CBT: Levels of Cognitive Processing

FIGURE 8.3   *Worksheet linking overt with covert dysfunctional beliefs*

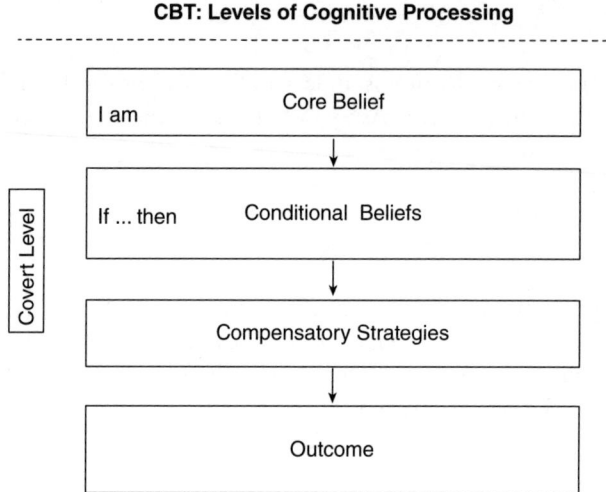

FIGURE 8.4 *Covert level of processing errors in Beck's psychopathology model*

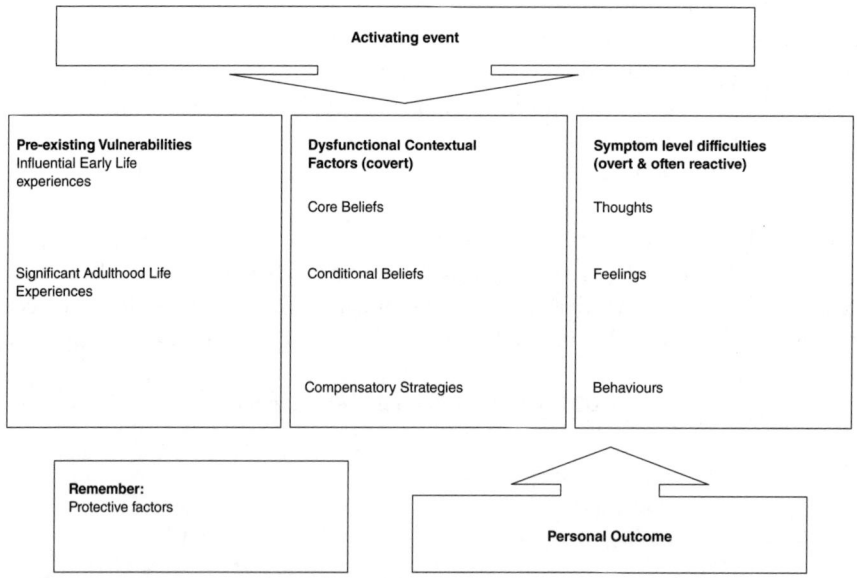

FIGURE 8.5 *Beck's model of psychopathology: conceptualization worksheet*

A copy of this figure is available to download from https://study.sagepub.com/laidlaw

In older people, the persistent and recurrent nature of presenting problems within the individual's own lifespan development may result in the development of a maladaptive schemata linked to a sense of failure and incompetence rendering the individual vulnerable and prone to the development of depression. As may be observed in the conceptualisation worksheet in Figure 8.5, unhelpful beliefs or rules for living are acknowledged as being likely to have their roots in adulthood experiences as much as in childhood ones. Hence, one must ask about experiences across the age span and not just in childhood, as one might do when working with adults of working age.

> Early experiences can be misunderstood to mean childhood or adolescent experiences when creating a conceptualisation with older people. This is too narrow. Over the course of a lifetime an individual may have experienced many significant life events that have changed the individual's view of self. Thus, early experiences occur across an entire life history of an individual and are *not* confined to early adulthood.

It is also evident in the model of psychopathology, and reflected in the Figure 8.5, that problems can occur at two levels: overt and covert (Persons, 1989). The overt level may reflect the reasons the person seeks therapy in the first place, so we can detect and measure overt symptomatology in depression through the thoughts, behaviours and emotions exhibited by the client. The covert level is less clear-cut, and reflects what Persons (1989) calls the 'underlying psychological mechanism'. The covert level reflects the dysfunctional, rigid schemata level of belief that undermines an individual in their attempts to manage their difficulties. Persons (2008) notes that multiple problems may stem from a single underlying psychological mechanism, or that there could be multiple mechanisms, although for reasons of practicality and simplicity it is important to restrain the number of underlying psychological mechanisms that are hypothesised in order to link the overt nature of problems with their underlying maintenance factors (Persons, 2008). It is this which explains the appraisals an individual is prone to make about situation or stressors. The Stoic philosopher Epictetus noted that a 'situation is neither good nor bad, but thinking makes it so'.

As case conceptualisation is a theory-driven action it can be delineated in specific detail. As you set out to contextualise your client's problems or challenges you may wish to be on the lookout for themes in the content of sessions and messages the individual gives themselves.

Multiple Levels of Conceptualisation

Case conceptualisation can occur at a number of levels and it isn't always necessary to string a complex set of 'boxes' together when more simple models of understanding are sufficient to explain a recurring pattern to the client.

Conceptualisation can occur most simply in terms of an interactive four-components model (also commonly known as the hot cross bun model, see Padesky & Mooney, 1990) identified in Figure 8.6.

In this model we might want to add in an additional factor such as the environment (meaning where the situation occurred and including the interactional style with significant others) when looking at how we can help people. This model simply and effectively aims to introduce clients to the idea that our thoughts are connected to feelings and

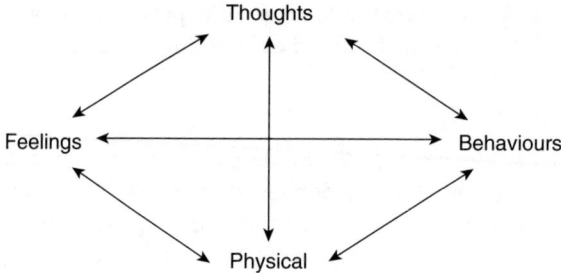

FIGURE 8.6   *The hot cross bun model for conceptualisation*

behaviour, and that we often experience a physical reaction at times of distress. At its most basic we can see that the four-components model within CBT functions pretty well as a very focused mini case-conceptualisation diagram, as it links thoughts, feelings, behaviours and physical states/symptoms in a reinforcing loop that is very effective at explaining how each element can contribute its own unique variance when considering a response to an experience. Its simplicity is a great strength, as it will not take a whole session to explain to a client and it can be used as a homework exercise to see if the client can identify other negatively reinforcing loops in their interaction with the world.

A four-components model is much easier to do when you have a context or a situation that produces stimulus response relationships. You may also note that the elements of this model are very much based in the here and now, but that often data emerge to indicate that there is a historical aspect to the experience that amplifies and accelerates the generation of negative affect and appraisal. The four-components model can also be augmented with an age-appropriate context as illustrated in Figure 7.6 (page 110).

A worked example using this type of framework (that also functions as a good way to socialise people to CBT) is available in Chapter 5 of this book (p. 70).

There are various ways to understand and use the different levels of conceptualisation. Mrs Tullibody is an 86-year-old widow who would habitually call herself names in therapy. The therapist noted that she often castigated herself about situations that in reality she handled with great diligence and skill. She would say she was stupid, mean and inadequate: 'I'm such a stupid girl'. She appeared to accept these bullying statements as factual and largely unworthy of challenge. The therapist recorded how often she would call herself such names. The therapist brought this information to the client's attention so that she was able to see how she undermined her self-confidence and esteem in ways that she would not dream of doing to others. The therapist used this name calling as an opportunity to discuss a simple conceptualisation within the session. The client had a history where after the death of her parents when she was aged nine, she went to live with two maiden aunts. This client had always been interested in the arts, particularly music and dance. Unfortunately, this was not a good match with her maiden aunts' interests who were more focused on science and the classics. The client is a talented pianist but she did not have an interest in science, and this led to her aunts castigating her for her poor performance in these subjects at the same time as ignoring the things she was good at. When the client and therapist worked together to make sense of her habitual statements, the client stated they were very similar to the comments her aunts made when she was young and was quickly able to distance herself from such comments. No cognitive restructuring was necessary as this was not a negative cognition as such, but more a product of an internalised negative schemata. The quick conceptualisation here is that early experiences have led to this client accepting uncritically the self-endorsed view of her by others. Thus, a process could be identified by the client using the formulation summary sheet in Figure 8.7.

This understanding was sufficient for the client to be motivated to adopt a different, more compassionate view. She noted that she did not use any 'parenting tips' when bringing up her own children and her main lesson was to let her children feel loved and to be able to be free to be themselves and pursue their own interests. Thus, in a compassionate self-strategy she was able to say that her aunt's view of her as a 'stupid girl' was neither factual nor helpful, that and she would challenge this statement in future.

Using the Client's Own Models of Understanding to Conceptualise Difficulties

The idiosyncratic nature of the way people make sense of things can be understood by looking at their thoughts, feelings and behaviours, and can provide insights that

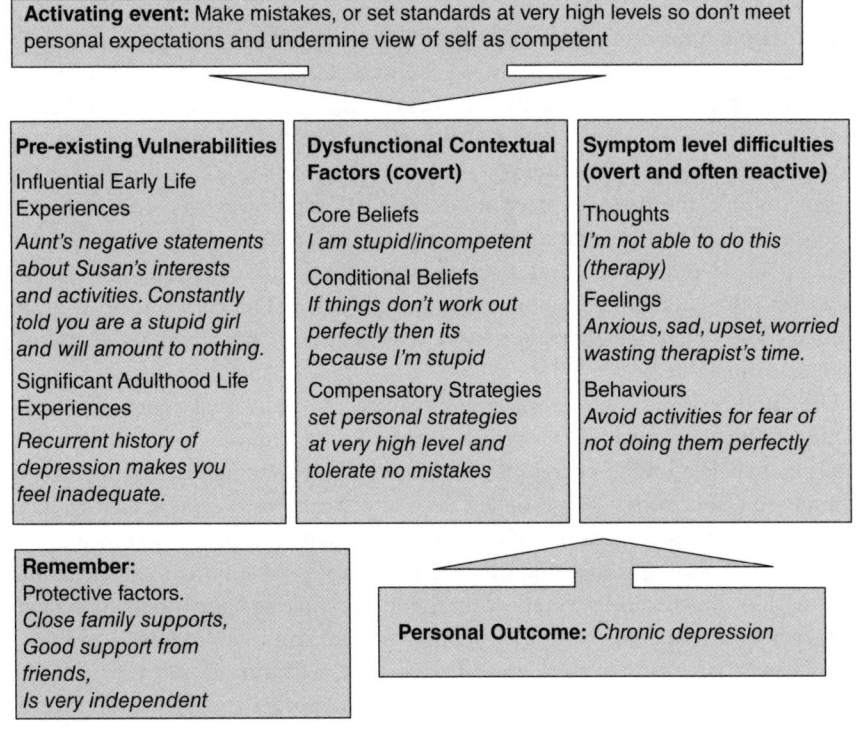

FIGURE 8.7 *Example of simple conceptualization*

are important in developing conceptualisations. These insights do not need to be the result of full conceptualisations, but can be gained from simpler ways of making sense of data presented within treatment.

A case conceptualisation also provides you with a way of seeing the bigger picture. Thus the conceptualisation allows us to *describe* the current problems and to make *predictions* about future events. Importantly they also point to *interventions* to avoid future distress.

Age-Appropriate CBT?

Sometimes CBT is criticised by practitioners as having too narrow a focus in its consideration of the problems older people bring into the clinic room. The use of a contextualising CBT framework that takes account of the bigger picture is presented below.

Meta-Competent Case Conceptualisation with Older People: Comprehensive Conceptualisation Framework for CBT with Older People

Sometimes there may be a need to consider conceptualising therapy within an age-appropriate frame of reference, so as to potentiate CBT's efficacy with older people. The Comprehensive Conceptualisation Framework (CCF, see Laidlaw et al., 2004) for CBT with older people, helps therapists, particularly those inexperienced in working with older people, provide a way of framing or contextualising older adults' problems within the standard Beck model of CBT. The main elements of the CCF are cohort beliefs, transition in role-investments, intergenerational linkages, the socio-cultural context and health status. Each element serves to broaden the understanding that a therapist will draw on when working with elders. The CCF model is outlined in much more detail elsewhere (see Laidlaw et al., 2004), but the main elements are summarised in Table 8.1.

The CCF provides a means of contextualising an individual's current set of difficulties within a lifespan developmental perspective. For example, taking account of cohort beliefs allows a therapist to acknowledge that different generations have different experiences that shape their values and world view, and as such these may have changed across generations. Knight (2004) emphasises that working with older people entails learning something of the folkways of people born many years previously. In order for therapists to reflect on the importance of cohort beliefs and values, consider the current cohort of older people who are true age pioneers.

For many older people who enter therapy, the activating event may indicate an unwanted transitions in role-investment, such as becoming the primary carer for one's spouse who has developed dementia. Alternatively, as one develops disability and loses independence this can be a painful and difficult transition for individuals to make (Broomfield et al., 2011).

TABLE 8.1 *Comprehensive Conceptualisation Framework (CCF) for CBT with older people (Laidlaw et al., 2004)*

Element of CCF	Description of CCF element	Clinical relevance
Cohort beliefs	Generational beliefs held by people born in similar years or at similar time periods that may determine values of these individuals across generations.	Cohort beliefs and values provide the context in which beliefs at a wider, more societal level can be understood. Thus, stigma about depression in older people may be understood at a cohort level. Cohort beliefs of older generations can also sometimes clash with the therapist's beliefs. For example, beliefs about lifestyle choices and gender roles may differ markedly, making therapists feel uncomfortable.
Intergenerational linkages	Within families there are different generations that come into regular contact. The different generations have different needs and outlooks. There may be opportunities for sharing of family values across generations and there may be opportunities for generativity where an older generation may help a younger generation share in wisdom of experience.	Intergenerational relationships may provoke tensions. If older people feel their views are being ignored or they are being marginalised because they are old this can cause tensions within the family. Likewise, if older people have previously cared for their 'elderly relatives' when younger they may adhere to beliefs of filial care that are not shared by other members of their family. Carers and care recipients may also develop intergenerational negative linkages. Older people in receipt of care may experience distress as they feel a 'burden' on their family.
Socio-cultural context	Depressed older people may state that their problems are to do with ageing. Healthcare professionals may also be seduced into the 'fallacy of good reasons' (Unutzer et al., 1999), believing such statements are factual and realistic appraisals of a difficult time of life. Levy (2009) has developed a theory of negative age stereotypes becoming self-stereotypes that can impact upon an individual in terms of affect, cognition, behaviour and physiology.	Many older people have an implicit assumption (that can be challenged with cognitive restructuring techniques) that old age inevitably means loss and decrepitude. In CBT internalised negative age stereotypes can be considered to be a latent and maladaptive vulnerability about ageing that has been reinforced and often endorsed by themselves and society for decades. Levy (2009) suggests negative societal attitudes about age are internalised from a very young age, and reinforced throughout adulthood by an attentional bias to negative information about ageing. Stereotypes internalised during childhood become self-stereotypes that function as predisposing vulnerabilities for development of negative attitudes to ageing. A possible mechanism for the activation of negative age stereotypes predicting and determining attitudes to ageing can be found by

(Continued)

TABLE 8.1 *(Continued)*

Element of CCF	Description of CCF element	Clinical relevance
		considering a stress–diathesis interaction. As individuals age, negative age stereotypes operating outside the individual's conscious awareness, become activated by congruent negative experiences attributed to ageing. Stated simply, negative events are attributed to the ageing process, and this explanatory construct reinforces individual negative appraisals congruent with the self-stereotype, suggesting an unpleasant experience of ageing is the norm. Depressed older people endorse negative attitudes to ageing that are plausible, distorted and unhelpful and may be accepted by the healthcare professionals they come in contact with. Older people who selectively attend to negative indicators of aging such as loss due to bereavement, or physical health changes such as a longstanding limiting non-life-threatening condition, may be more prone to activations of the internalised negative age stereotype (the diathesis). The socio-cultural context also takes into account the values of the therapist.
Transitions in role investments	The transitions in role investment experienced by people are important variables to consider when working with older people. In later life there may be transitions that an individual needs to navigate in order to adapt successfully to age-related changes. Common transitions that may be challenging are becoming a primary caregiver for a loved one, or transitioning to living alone. For many older people experiencing the bereavement of their partner means they may be experiencing living alone for the first time in many years, and for some this is the first experience of this in their adult lives.	Transitions in role investments commonly seen in later life can become problematic when people attempt to cope with a change in circumstances by rigidly and inflexibly adhering to outmoded coping strategies that in the past served them well. Examples of transitions in role investments with the potential for distress are when an individual loses independence because of a change in physical health status, or when taking on a new role such as caregiving. The amount of investment one has in the roles that give life personal meaning may be an important determinant in how successfully one adapts to a changed circumstance.

Element of CCF	Description of CCF element	Clinical relevance
Health status	Increasing age brings with it an increased likelihood of developing chronic medical conditions. Ill health can be understood in terms of three components: impairment, disability and handicap (WHO, 1980):	CBT therapists can usefully employ elements of the Baltes model of selection optimisation with compensation (SOC; Freund & Baltes, 1998) approach to optimal ageing (see Laidlaw & Pachana, 2009). Highly valued roles and goals are maintained as older people select alternative means of achieving these goals.
	• Impairment refers to the loss or abnormality of body structure, appearance, organ or system (e.g. infarct in a stroke).	Selection (usually 'loss-based selection') is a process where highly valued roles and goals are maintained in the face of loss where an individual modifies goal-attainment due to a reduction in resources.
	• Disability is the impact of the impairment (e.g. infarct in a certain part of a person's brain) on the individual's ability to carry out 'normal' activities.	Optimisation requires that an individual focus resources on achieving goals through the practising or relearning of activities. It must be done in an intentional manner. Compensation requires that an individual engage in alternative means of achieving the highest possible level of functioning, therefore taking account of the reality of a person's capacity and physical integrity.
	• Handicap can be thought of as the social impact that the impairment or disease has on the individual. Consequences of handicap are visible when a person interacts with his or her environment. Thus, a person who has experienced a stroke may find that other people now treat them differently, by excluding him or her from normal communications.	SOC can be incorporated into psychotherapy, especially CBT, as the problem-solving orientation is a good fit with an aim of symptom reduction and achievement of an improvement in functioning. The usefulness of the WHO (1980) classification to therapists is that it allows one to consider an individual's impairment or disease simply and to separate out the consequences from the impairment. CBT works at the level of disability and handicap, but not at the level of impairment. An alternative is to use the later WHO ICF framework as a way to incorporate health factors.

Cohort

Cohort can be understood simply as values and beliefs shared amongst a generational group of individuals born at a similar time period. Taking account of cohort beliefs, allows a therapist to acknowledge different generations have different experiences that shape their values.
Relevant Gero-Theory: Socio-emotional Selectivity Theory (Carstensen et al., 1999).

Transitions in Role Investments

The changes and adaptations older people may have to consider to maintain activities and interests that are personally meaningful and relevant to an individual valuation of quality of life. This may be the point at which a person starts to notice age related challenges.
Relevant Gero-Theory:
Diehl & Werner-Wahl, (2010) Awarness of Age Related Change.

Early Experiences

Idiosycratically important events that can occur throughout the lifespan and includes significant Adult Life events information of schemata

Core Beliefs
Rigid and dysfunctional fixed beliefs

Activating Events
Stressors that predispose a person to develop distress

Conditional Beliefs/Underlying Assumptions
Idiosyncratic rules governing behaviour with cognition and emotional consequences often stated in 'if...then' conditional terms

Compensatory Strategies
Coping strategies and mechanisms that allow an individual to function in the world despite dysfunctional cognitions, attitudes and behaviour.

Negative Automatic Thoughts
Content of a person's thoughts reflecting negative cognitive 'trait': self, world, future

DEPRESSION

Cognitive *Affective*

Physiological *Behavioural*

Intergenerational Linkages

The importance of family and the transmission of idiosyncratic family values. The importance of generativity from one generation to the next. This has the potential for positive as well as negative consequences for the client.
Relevant Gero-Theory:
Socio-emotional Selectivity Theory (Carstensen et al., 1999). Antonucci's Convoy Model.

Socio-cultural Context

The internalisation of societal level beliefs about ageing and older people. Older people often reject association with their in-group. May be assessed with the Attitudes to Ageing Questionnaire, especially psycho-social loss.
Relevant Gero-Theory:
Levy (2009) Stereotype Embodiment theory of the internalisation of the negative age stereotype.

Health status: The impact of health conditions that can be understood at an individual level either by understanding the interaction of impairment, disability or handicap or by reference to the WHO international classification of functioning, disability and health (ICF) taking account of body factors, societal and individual perspectives and the environment.
The strategies that may assist an individual to effectively manage the impact of a potentially limiting chronic and/or deteriorating condition are summarized by the use of Selection, Optimisation with Compensation (Freund and Baltes, 1998).

Comprehensive Cognitive Formulation for CBT with Older People (CCF): Laidlaw et al., 2004

FIGURE 8.8 *The key elements of the Comprehensive Conceptualization Framework*

Within the CCF, each individual is considered to be constantly striving to achieve homeostasis throughout his or her life trajectory. People come into therapy because of transitions in circumstance that are proving hard to navigate alone, with recourse to habitual strategies, and the CCF helps therapists contextualise problems within an age-appropriate frame of reference that retains the treatment focus of a CBT formulation. The key elements of the CCF are illustrated in Figure 8.8 and the case example that follows.

Case Example: Harry

Harry is a 68-year-old retired engineer. He has been referred by his GP because of chronic low mood. His doctor has tried Harry on a number of medications, but the side effects have proven difficult for Harry to tolerate. Harry has returned 'home' after working in Kenya for most of his life. He and his wife live alone in a cottage in a small rural town in Scotland. He states that his mood is often low because of the poor weather. He has found it difficult to settle in the UK and he often contemplates returning to Kenya. He has tried to get involved in voluntary work but nothing has been available to utilise his skills; a local college were keen to have him lecture on troubleshooting in engineering, but they decided against employing him because he is beyond retirement age. He says he feels 'rootless and useless'.

Harry also considers himself 'foolish for coming back home'. He thinks he would have been much better off if he had stayed and worked in the UK rather than emigrating in the late 1960s as his pension would now be better. He compares himself unfavourably with other men he 'left behind' many years ago. Harry has two sons still living in Kenya. His youngest son is going through a messy divorce and Harry feels depressed that this is happening. He thinks he has failed his children. He says that 'If we had stayed I might have been able to help . . . I might have prevented the divorce [of my son].' The therapist asked Harry to give evidence for this belief and then evidence against. The information provided is presented in Table 8.2.

After this exercise, Harry can see that the evidence-against column is compelling. When the therapist asks Harry to reflect on the circumstances around the divorce of his eldest son, he sees that he has been thinking in rigid ways. This also seems to be further evidence to Harry that he lost another role that he considers important. He also feels angry that his son doesn't seem to 'need' him anymore.

TABLE 8.2   *Evidence for and against Harry's beliefs*

Evidence for (staying would have helped)	Evidence against
Getting kids at weekend may have relieved the pressure	He only wants help when he feels ready and I can't force him to accept my help
I could have been someone to talk to	He might see me as being interfering – there
I could have given him confidence – he needs support	is a fine line between interfering and helping
	I might have been too close if I had stayed
I could have been someone for him to fall back on	Maybe if we had still been living in __ it would have made it (separation) more likely as he could have fallen back on us

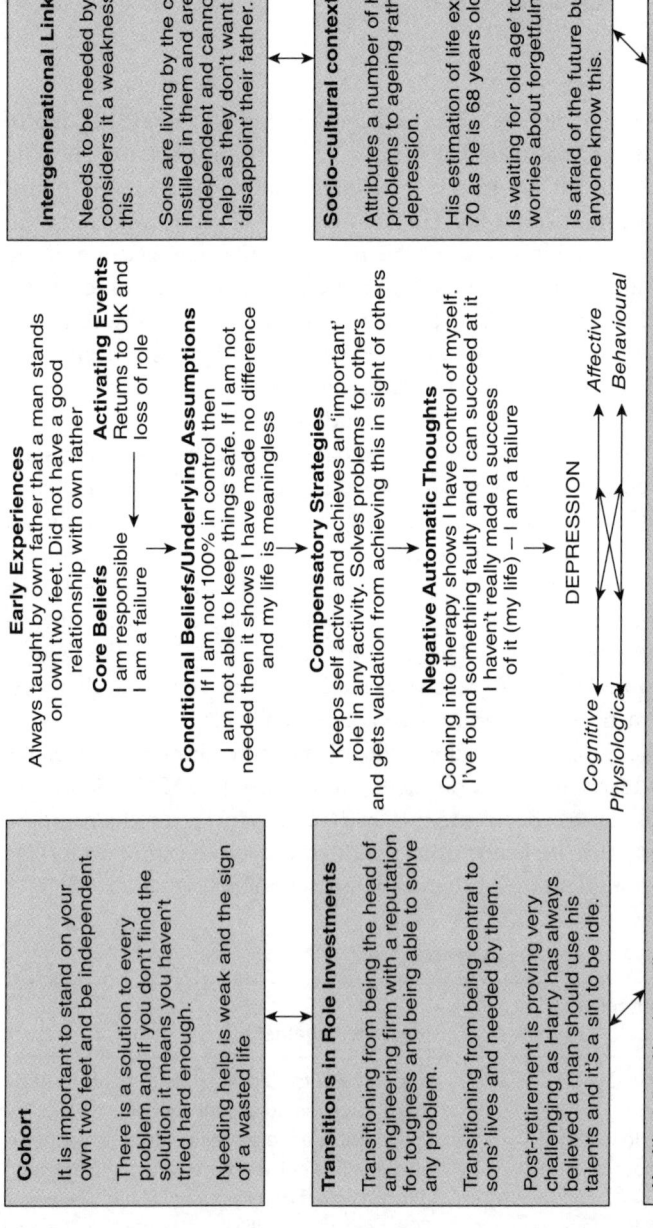

FIGURE 8.9 *Diagrammatic conceptualisation of the CCF for Harry*

A blank copy of this figure is available to download from https://study.sagepub.com/laidlaw

TABLE 8.3 *Conceptualisation Reflection Worksheet*

I found this aspect of the conceptualisation easier to do	I found this aspect of the conceptualisation more difficult to do

Learning task for myself:

A copy of this table is available to download from https://study.sagepub.com/laidlaw

Harry dislikes being in therapy as he was always taught he should stand on his own two feet. He says that 'By coming here I'm not in control of myself,' and 'I am being disloyal to my family by discussing problems here.'

He has high expectations for a rapid improvement in his mood, and apart from his depression was in good health until he was diagnosed with type 2 diabetes. This came as quite a shock as he had kept himself fit and active and did not consider himself particularly overweight. He said that when his hair started to go he hated it but he coped, but now with 'old people's illnesses' starting to affect him, he is worried that he'll become decrepit and old. 'I hate the thought of growing old' he says. Figure 8.9 provides a diagrammatic conceptualisation of the CCF for Harry.

Summary

Conceptualisation in CBT with older people can occur at many different levels, and for it to be helpful in therapy it need not be especially complex. Sometimes there is a need to contextualise CBT work with older people in an age-appropriate context. Case conceptualisation is a skill that can be honed, and makes more sense the more you do it. It may not be easy at first as it involves learning a whole set of terminology and may also require you to think about clinical data in a different way. It may also be challenging to try to summarise all your ideas about the nature of your client and how it is that they struggle with their problems in the way that they do. To simplify things, perhaps you can ask yourself: 'what are the meanings of events from the client's point of view that make this situation more painful/challenging/distressing for them?' It may be useful for you to take a moment to reflect on what aspects of conceptualisations are difficult for you (see Table 8.3).

Learning Log: Reflection and Review
What have you gained from reading this chapter?

- Think of a case you are working on right now. Can you use the ideas here to develop a case conceptualisation?
- Taking a case you know very well, think about the gaps in the worksheet you may have.

(Continued)

(Continued)

- Choose a case you know very well and think about the different levels of conceptualisation and how this idea would work for you in practice.
- Decide for yourself what the advantages are for each of the three main conceptualisation frameworks when working with older people, and make a mental list of their advantages. Try out each framework with a case you know well and consider what added value is derived from their use.

Further Reading

The following sources provide more in-depth coverage of topics raised in this chapter.

Kuyken, W., Padesky, C. A., & Dudley, R. (2009). *Collaborative case conceptualization: working effectively with clients in cognitive behavioral therapy*. New York: Guilford Press.

Laidlaw, K., Thompson, L., & Gallagher-Thompson, D. (2004). Comprehensive conceptualisation of cognitive behaviour therapy for late life depression, *Behavioural & Cognitive Psychotherapy, 32*, 1–11.

Persons, J. B. (2008). *The case formulation approach to cognitive-behavior therapy*. New York: Guilford Press.

PART 3
Specialist Applications of CBT with Older People

Nine

Augmented Age-Appropriate CBT: Enhancing Wisdom, Resilience and Self-Acceptance

Learning Objectives

By the end of this chapter you will:

- Understand the value of gerontology as a good source of information to understand the modern experience of ageing
- Appreciate how to use timelines when working with older people with depression and anxiety
- Be able to augment CBT outcome by helping clients use their own experiences of coping with events/overcoming adversity to help them deal with the here-and-now problems they present with, and to cope better in the future by becoming resilient and self-accepting

A New Framework for CBT with Older People

In older people, the persistent and recurrent nature of presenting problems within an individual's own lifespan development may create an idiosyncratic, unhelpful narrative of failure and incompetence, rendering the individual vulnerable to the development of chronic anxiety and depression symptoms. The emotional and cognitive consequences of experiences throughout a lifespan may continue to shape latent maladaptive schemata throughout adulthood. A stress–diathesis for the development of depression or anxiety in later life must therefore take account of proximal as well as distal experiences when understanding an individual's vulnerabilities in the context of possible treatment interventions. Hence, therapists need to ask about experiences across the lifespan and not just in childhood, as one might do when working with adults of working age.

Currently, therapists working with older people have limited age-appropriate psychological treatment models that characterise the complexity and chronicity of problems that older people bring to therapy. Changes made to CBT approaches by individual clinicians run the risk of diluting the focus of CBT, and may also promote therapeutic drift (Waller, 2009).

Gerontology – the science of ageing, as opposed to geriatrics – may hold the key to augmenting CBT such that it meets the needs of older people. Therapists may wish to appraise themselves of gerontological theories of emotional regulation, which suggest that older people become more skilled in this domain as they age (Scheibe & Carstensen, 2010). Similarly, theories of wisdom in older people also present a potentially useful perspective for CBT therapists on how to use life experiences (Staudinger & Glück, 2011). Selective optimisation with compensation (SOC) (Chapter 10) and age stereotypes in CBT (Chapter 7) are further examples of the usefulness of applied gerontology for CBT therapists working with older people.

As CBT has been shown to be an efficacious treatment, changes can only be justified if they potentially enhance treatment outcome. At the same time, variability in the experience of ageing and the heterogeneity of this population (Zeiss & Steffen, 1996) suggest that modifications of therapeutic procedures may not always be necessary. Laidlaw et al. (2004) developed an age-appropriate contextualisation framework for CBT with older people to help therapists understand their clients' problems more broadly (see Chapter 8).

Wisdom Enhancement in CBT with Older People

Wisdom is an important theoretical gerontological concept that could provide a positive frame of reference for affective change in CBT with older people (Knight & Laidlaw, 2009). Consistent with the active goal-directed perspective of CBT, 'The acquisition of an expert system of wisdom . . . requires concerted personal and societal investment of considerable time, effort, motivation, and structured experience' (Baltes & Smith, 2008: 58). Thus, CBT can precipitate gains in wisdom and wisdom can augment treatment outcome.

Wisdom retains an allure among many people (Laidlaw, 2013b). It functions as a commonly understood 'folk theory' emphasising growth with advancing age (Bluck & Glück, 2004). However, wisdom is rarely simply an outcome of age (Staudinger & Glück, 2011). Wisdom at an individual level may be more likely to develop through individuals becoming adept at navigating uncertainty and ambiguity over a lifetime of experiences (Laidlaw, 2013a). Personal wisdom therefore depends on learning from experience, but may also be evident in judicious actions in ambiguous situations (Sternberg, 2012). The concept of wisdom enhancement in CBT is a relatively simple one and is summarised in Figure 9.1.

An interesting parallel between wisdom and psychotherapy can be found in studies indexing wise actions. When individuals are asked to respond to dilemmas on their own, wise answers are impoverished compared to responses generated in discussion with significant others or in groups, or when individuals are directed to consult an 'inner voice' (Baltes and Staudinger, 2000). This is analogous to the experience of therapy, in that a 'problem shared is a problem halved'. Therapy sessions can therefore

Basically the idea of wisdom enhancement in CBT is a simple one.

1. When people are depressed autobiographical memory is overgeneralised and vague

2. Mood-congruent biases and the tendency to ruminate in depression will block wisdom-attainment (learning from and using past experience)

3. Resulting in long term vulnerability and chronicity

- Thus older people will look back upon a life history and selectively evaluate their life history in terms of failure
- In CBT the emphasis is 'here and now'
- A life lived will be full of ups and downs and we need to make use of that rich data in CBT when working with older people
- We use the life experience to help individuals deal better with current dilemmas/problems
- It is a valuing and respectful application of CBT for use with older people. It ought to work equally well with people who have an experience of chronic depression with multiple episodes of depression.

FIGURE 9.1 *Wisdom Enhancement Principles applied to CBT*

provide a nurturing environment for the growth of wisdom. As Baltes and Smith (2008: 62) comment 'For example, people can be guided to express markedly higher levels of wisdom-related knowledge by memory cues or instructions to consult an inner voiced (internal dialogue with significant others). This may also be true when it comes to emotion regulation.'

For many, wisdom is the pinnacle of successful lifespan development and is highly valued in society (Staudinger & Glück, 2011). Thus, a CBT approach to enhance wisdom could be empowering to clients but also challenging, as many individuals in distress and besieged by negative cognitions may not find it easy to consider themselves in possession of such a valued construct.

Baltes and Staudinger (2000) define five criteria as the means of assessing wisdom behaviours: rich factual and procedural knowledge, which is about 'knowing what' as well as 'knowing how' in the execution of decisions and activities; accrual of experience across a lifetime informs a self-identity; the relativism of values and priorities (lifespan contextualism); and how an individual deals with the recognition and management of uncertainty.

The Baltes wisdom model corresponds very well with the experience of older people participating in CBT, as they value use of experience and recommend think aloud protocols when dealing with complex problems (Baltes & Kunzmann, 2004). When someone comes into treatment in CBT their idiosyncratic way of seeing the world and understanding their problems is analogous to lifespan contextualism. In order for therapy to proceed, the therapist and client must agree on a shared sense of priorities and goals, and this is similar to the concept of relativism of values and priorities. Also, a person often comes into therapy because of a transition that is proving difficult in one way or another, and where there is no obvious solution. Sometimes for therapy to proceed it is simply necessary for the client to understand that a decision is neither good nor bad, it is just a decision. In this case it is similar to the recognition and management of uncertainty.

As can be pointed out, wisdom is about recognising the nature of life and the impossibility of living a life free from mistakes, complexity and compromises. Wisdom can therefore foster self-forgiveness and acceptance (Germer & Siegel, 2012). In this domain, wisdom enhancement in CBT has the potential for improving the quality of life of clients beyond symptom reduction. 'Wisdom, as measured by our paradigm, goes hand in hand with balance, modulation, and the ability to distance oneself from difficult situations, if this is considered functional' (Baltes & Kunzmann, 2004: 296). This description of wisdom attainment provides a clear connection with a CBT approach.

Augmenting CBT with Older People?

A logical approach to augmenting CBT treatment is to consider what differences there may be in working with older people. The first obvious difference is that older people have many more life experiences to bring into therapy. CBT recognises that clients bring a rich factual and procedural knowledge with them. In CBT with older people we do not always have to teach clients new skills, we simply need to remind individuals to use their pre-existing skills and competences. Older people seen in our clinics are survivors. They have survived past setbacks, survived past episodes of depression and anxiety, and have overcome adversity that younger therapists may have not yet faced (Laidlaw, 2013b).

Working with older people who may have a recurrent history of depression and/or anxiety may present problems when trying to take a history of the client and in agreeing how to overcome problems. However, CBT provides the means by which clients can put their past history under the microscope in order to discover more about themselves and to learn from past mistakes. Overgeneralised, vague attributions about past events are unlikely to provide much in the way of constructive learning opportunities. Watkins et al. (2009) demonstrate how to teach depressed people to become 'concrete thinkers' with reduced symptoms of depression and reduced levels of self-criticism.

While ageing offers numerous experiences of life and ample opportunity to develop wisdom, clearly not everyone learns from their experiences. Depression may block wisdom attainment because of the selective and overgeneralised nature of recall in depression and the excessively negative attributions an individual makes about themselves (Joorman et al., 2009). Negative affect increases accessibility of mood congruent material (Gotlib & Joorman, 2010) with a potential for a false positive recall for negative information (Joorman et al., 2009). Therefore, an individual may find it hard to find positives when recalling the past. This selective recall may also be seen when older people fail to use their lifetime experience to help them deal with their fears (Laidlaw, 2010a). For example, Mrs Alwyn is an 81-year-old widower. She worries constantly about her adult children and grandchildren and is currently worried about the health of her sister. She is afraid that if her sister's condition worsens she will be unable to cope (her sister has diabetes). She says with absolute certainty that her biggest fear is the death of her sister, as she fears that she would not cope without her weekly visits from her sister.

The therapist was aware that Mrs Alwyn had lost her husband to cancer two years previously after forty-eight years of marriage. This had been an exceptionally difficult experience for Mrs Alwyn, who described it as the worst event of her life and the realisation of her worst fears. Thus, when talking with Mrs Alwyn about her fears about her sister, the therapist asked his client if she had ever had to face her worst fear. Mrs Alwyn initially said she hadn't, but when she was reminded of her struggle and eventual mastery of coping after the very great loss of her husband, she acknowledged that she was a lot stronger than she gave herself credit for. In examining how resilient she is in reality the therapist asked Mrs Alwyn to review how she had coped since her husband had died. Achievements she could identify were listed as follows: she was living alone in a house for the first time in her life, she was independent and proud of herself for fixing her own fuses, and she started dancing just after her husband died and participated in dance shows. Recently a friend of her husband's had died and for the first time she went to a funeral on her own, saying 'Wow, I am amazed at myself. From someone who never even went to funerals. I now cope on my own. Very proud of that.'

The important thing to take from this example is how resilient older people are. For Mrs Alwyn her experience of therapy success is likely to be integrated into her personal life narrative that she constructs, integrating her values, defining memories and low and high points in her life, termed 'personal myths' (McAdams & Adler, 2010). People construct personal narratives as a way of giving meaning to their life and experiences (McAdams, 2001). For therapists working with clients using CBT it should be evident that the veracity of personal myths are not important as the meaning that is attached to them, and therapists can use this as a vehicle for change towards resilience.

The gains made by Mrs Alwyn can also be seen as evidence that she is able to reflect upon and reframe narratives associated with past experiences in a way that promotes growth (Bauer & McAdams, 2004). In her narrative she has created a sense of agency consistent with wisdom enhancement following CBT. Narratives that are associated with positive outcomes after adversity are linked to enhanced well-being (McAdams & Adler, 2010).

Use the Wisdom of Years: Using the Past to Help One Cope with the Present

Wisdom can also be enhanced by explicitly asking people to reflect on difficult life experiences in a highly structured way to see if they can differentiate a range of outcomes (good and bad) from difficult experiences from the past, and identify whether these experiences have some value for the client. By adopting this approach – of seeing past life challenges as opportunities for growth – a normalising strategy is adopted, in that clients are encouraged to see challenges as part of life. This is also destigmatising, as surviving challenging circumstances may have required emotional regulation, and the individual may have coped with the situation as best they could at the time. The narrative is that they have survived difficulties and may be changed after the experience. McAdams (2006) talks of individuals developing 'redemptive sequences' where a bad experience or event can be transformed into a growth experience by the individual.

Stripped to its psychological essence, redemption is the deliverance from suffering to an enhanced status, or state. In life stories, redemptive sequences begin with the protagonist's experience of a negative emotional state such as fear, guilt, shame or despair. The negative scene, however, gives way to the

experience of happiness, joy, excitement, growth or some other positive emotional state. (McAdams, 2006: 88)

Resilience shares some positive and valued attributes with wisdom, in that individuals who are better endowed in these areas are more able to cope with adversity
and may also be better able to deal with challenges with greater flexibility as opposed
to falling back on rigid habits that are no longer fit for purpose. The difference
between wisdom and resilience is that individuals who are resilient draw upon this
resource when faced with adversity without the need for too much reflection. Wise
individuals, on the other hand, understand the value of using past experience in order
to better meet new challenges – they are able to deal with ambiguity by recognising
the similarities and differences in challenges they face, and being able to discriminate
between possible coping strategies.

Helping the individual to recognise their resilience in the face of difficult circumstances can be used to help the person deal with the 'here and now' in dealing with
anxiety or depression. To promote this thinking the therapist may ask the individual:
'What is a wise thing to do. Using the wisdom of your years' (Knight & Laidlaw,
2009), when discussing how to proceed with ambiguous and challenging circumstances. It is a Socratic discussion that is aimed at promoting an increased sense of
self-agency and the facilitation of focused problem-oriented thinking.

A clinical example of wisdom enhancement is Elsie coping with depressive hopelessness by reflecting on her experience in a concrete way. Elsie is a 71-year-old woman
with a recurrent history of depression stretching over her adult lifetime (see Laidlaw,
2010b). She has experienced at least six separate episodes of major depressive disorder
since her mid-20s. At the time of discussion, she had been admitted to hospital and had
lost hope about her future prospects for recovery. She said, 'I can't see me ever getting
back to how I used to be,' and 'I think I'll be in hospital for the rest of my life now.'

The therapist sought to elicit hope regarding the potential for change by asking
Elsie to use the 'wisdom of your experience with depression' (Laidlaw, 2010b). The
therapist introduced the idea that by having previous episodes of depression she
might be able to use those experiences to help her manage her current episode. It
was a conscious attempt to invoke a redemptive sequence to her negative past experiences. By being experienced with depression she was at an advantage in knowing that
symptoms resolve. The therapist asked Elsie: 'When you were depressed before, did
you ever think that you would not recover?' Elsie was able to see that she had thought
this in every previous episode of depression. The therapist sought to help Elsie process
this further by asking: 'So, what does that tell you?' Elsie said 'well maybe I was wrong
then and I'll be wrong this time'. The therapist asked Elsie if she thought this might
be possible, whereupon Elsie said 'I have this image in my head. I can see myself sitting in the ward in 1973, here in this hospital, and I'm staring out the window.' Elsie
recounted that she clearly remembered thinking that she would be in the ward for
the rest of her life. She recalled this as a vivid image. Elsie was able to use the vivid
sense of having experienced a conviction that recovery was not possible for her to
unseat some sense of her lack of recovery for her current episode. What made this
image all the more powerful is that Elsie made a full recovery and went on to marry
and have a child. None of these experiences seemed possible to her in the midst of

her depression, and these were powerful data for her to reflect on when experiencing her current sense of hopelessness and despair. While this intervention can be seen as cognitive restructuring, it is also a novel use in therapy of lifetime experiences to help an individual deal with a current challenge that appears unchangeable. It was also very empowering for Elsie to understand that she had answers to current difficulties by drawing on her own life experiences (Laidlaw, 2010b).

Wisdom Enhancement as a Target in CBT

Wisdom enhancement explicitly seeks to link people to their life experiences, and contextualises current episodes of distress within a lifespan perspective. Narrative approaches can be useful here, as personal stories that people construct continue over a lifetime are dynamic and open to reinterpretation – while they have connections with the past they need not be determined by it (McAdams & Adler, 2010). This implies that autobiographical memory is less fixed than might be supposed. Older clients seen in therapy who have experienced depression or anxiety over a number of episodes may have constructed a personal narrative of failure or personal misfortune. It may be reassuring for the therapist to understand that these seemingly fixed views are symptom-contaminated – change the symptoms and you change the narrative. Growth is therefore possible at any age.

A useful technique for the therapist to employ when understanding an individual's personal narrative is to ask them to construct a 'timeline' early on in therapy as a homework task. The timeline can be located on a vertical line that connects the individual's birthdate at the start of the timeline with the current date at the end of the timeline.

The therapist can ask the client to put all notable lifetime events on this timeline. The completion of the timeline is left to the client, although they can be based on overall life events, adverse life events, turning points (high or low) or a combination of all three. You could also ask the client to indicate 3–5 most significant life events on their timeline. Figure 9.2 illustrates what a timeline looks like.

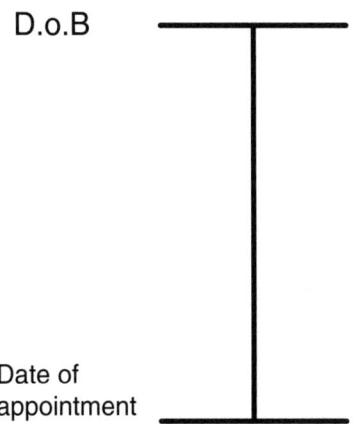

FIGURE 9.2   *Timeline in CBT*

By employing this simple technique the therapist gains an 'edited' summary of the high and low points of an individual's life. This technique can also save time, as it means you do not need to spend a long period gathering background information in the sessions and can use this for more active intervention. It is also interesting how clients approach the completion of this task. One client who was severely depressed and suicidal listed only negative events, and there was a total absence of positive or even neutral life events. The client was asked to complete another side to their timeline with significant positive events to be listed. This was a challenging task for her to complete, but in being directed to focus on this the client surprised herself by listing a number of positive events. Another client who had an event from her mid-life that she experienced great shame and sorrow over, completed a timeline with a significant time gap between 1973 and 1987. This allowed the therapist to explore her thoughts about this difficult time period in her life. Some clients have an approach that lists negative events on the left-hand side of the vertical line and positive events on the right-hand side. Figure 9.3 summarises principles in the application of timelines in CBT as follows:

- Step one: Develop a timeline (a good homework task?).
  - Look at timeline and acknowledge the strengths and resilience of the individual.
  - Does life's adversity make us wise? Can we define what we mean by wisdom?

- Step two: When examining past experience agree certain rules apply:
  - Reflection rather than blame – good and bad are part of life.
  - No hindsight bias on decisions made.

- Step three: Consider some experiences from the past.

- Step four: Is there a time in your client's life when they could be considered to have done something wise ... or when they coped with adversity?

- Step five: What can they learn from these times?
  - Enquire about what stops client from coping as well as they have in the past.

- Step six: Can these experiences they have handling ambiguous situations help them deal with current problems?

FIGURE 9.3   *Principles for using timelines in CBT with Older People*

It is in taking these elements from the timeline that wisdom enhancement comes into use. Jennifer (68 years old) was referred by her doctor and was given an explanation for her ongoing difficulties in terms of personality deficits – she was advised not to expect too many gains from treatment. She had a strong internalised view of herself as selfish and weak. Jennifer stated that 'During my life when things have gone wrong, instead of addressing them I've turned to help from others,' and 'What a mess I make of my life. I make these decisions and I can't cope with them.' Consequently, her default approach to managing challenges or problems was to seek an external 'rescue', as she did not have a strong sense of her own personal agency and ability to cope. This manifested itself most clearly at the start of therapy in her regular (daily) contact with the Samaritans helpline when she became upset. This erroneous view of self undermined Jennifer and resulted in prolonged contact with psychiatric services. From looking at her timeline, Jennifer has a tendency to make negative self-comparisons, in that she often appraises her actions as deficient in comparison to how she believes others would cope: 'I can't cope with anything, other people seem to manage much better about things than I do.' The therapist working with her stated he could not share her view of herself as weak. She had experienced many challenges in life and evidently had survived these as well as could be expected.

The therapist introduced the idea that Jennifer might wish to consider how she could use her experiences from her past in order to develop some wisdom for dealing with current difficulties. A new diary was introduced to support this intervention (see Figure 9.4).

Jennifer was constantly told she was incompetent and selfish from an early age. Despite this, she did well at school and was a sensitive and compassionate individual who liked to help others. Jennifer married and had two children, whom she has brought up in an atmosphere of unconditional love. Jennifer's husband died in mid-life, leaving her to struggle to bring up her children alone, and she did this by going back to work and providing for them. In mid-life, Jennifer developed breast cancer

Wisdom worksheet:

It is quite commonly thought that wisdom comes with age. Research evidence suggest otherwise. Usually it is challenging or difficult experiences that change us. It is those experiences that are difficult for us to navigate in life may help us at some point to become wiser after the event.

1. Think of a person you would consider wise. What was it that made you think of them? How would you describe them? What are their characteristics? What was it they did that made them wise in your eyes?
2. Now think back to a difficult situation in your life *(note if this causes you great distress, stop and distract yourself and we can discuss in our next session)*. It can be from the recent or more distant past. What did you do to help yourself cope? What was the outcome at the time? Looking back on it with the passing of time, what do you think about how you coped?
3. Now recall the wise person and try to imagine what they would have done in that situation? How differently would they do things from what you did? Looking back how differently would you do things now?

FIGURE 9.4 *Wisdom worksheet*

A copy of this figure is available to download from https://study.sagepub.com/laidlaw

and had a mastectomy. She has also experienced a number of other physical illnesses and has had to cope for a large part of her adult life on her own. Jennifer found it difficult to accept her depression symptoms, often seeing these as further evidence of her being self-indulgent, saying 'Along the way I have picked up that if you're depressed you must be a selfish person.' For many older people depression can be a shameful and painful experience because of how they perceive themselves. Some aspects of this self-view are linked with cohort beliefs for this generation (see Chapter 6).

From discussing experiences in the timeline it was evident that Jennifer was empathic and accepting of other people. Using cognitive distancing, Jennifer was able to stand back and view her experiences as if through the lens of another viewer, and began to challenge her self-view as incompetent, gradually replacing this with a cognitive reframing of herself as a resilient survivor.

The challenge in CBT is to ensure that clients become attuned to reframing past 'setbacks' in a more nuanced way, in order that they can recognise and acknowledge the internal resources they possess to optimise functioning in light of current problems and challenges. However, this work is challenging as it requires the client to become more self-compassionate and accepting. Compassion and understanding are often easier when it comes to others rather than oneself. It is easier to be compassionate to others as it makes one feel virtuous to act kindly towards our fellow man. Directed inwards, compassion and acceptance can feel uncomfortably self-indulgent and a cop-out (Laidlaw, 2013a).

Over the course of treatment there are many opportunities for setbacks, as recovery rarely proceeds in a linear positive direction. Self-punitive appraisals can undermine clients in their efforts to overcome depression and anxiety symptoms. Jennifer experienced a number of challenges during therapy treatment, as she often had unrealistic expectations for how she should manage situations. After recovering at home following a knee operation, Jennifer became anxious about the recovery she was making and consequently stopped engaging in constructive acts to manage her mood. She telephoned her therapist and tearfully exclaimed she had failed him and let him down, as she was feeling very low. She was greatly ashamed about how she was feeling. The therapist encouraged Jennifer to focus on what she could do in that moment to help herself feel better. Over the phone, Jennifer agreed a set of behavioural experiments to be completed as homework. She did these tasks to good effect. At the next appointment, the therapist and Jennifer focused on how it felt when she negatively self-evaluated herself for feeling unwell.

Her therapist advocated that she start to self-soothe by using positive affirmations as to how she was coping. Furthermore, she was encouraged to use compassionate self-acceptance (see Laidlaw, 2013a). She found this task difficult, as she was concerned that 'taking it easy' on herself when she was struggling was likely to mean she would end up in a worse position. She said, 'I'm frightened that too much [self] kindness would make me fold up,' and 'Being too kind/soft could have damaged my resolve.' The therapist used the timeline with Jennifer to review the pros and cons of self-criticism and self-acceptance (compassion) at times of crisis.

This became the focus of a new homework task: to contrast two ways of treating herself and to consider the emotional, cognitive and behavioural consequences of being hard on herself, or being compassionate when she was in distress. A self-acceptance diary was created for this process (see Figure 9.5).

Becoming a concrete thinker!

If you have recently been experiencing distress about a situation or event and you've noticed that you've been blaming yourself in a overgeneral way, e.g. 'Why do I always do this', perhaps it may be useful to try a few steps to help you become more compassionate (kinder) towards yourself.

Remembering that when we are struggling or are in pain, it doesn't help to chastise ourselves, it only makes us more depressed and feeling less in control. It becomes demotivating. If you are not sure of this think about the pros and cons of being hard/strict versus kind/compassionate toward yourself:

Advantages of being hard on self	Disadvantages at time of stress/distress

In the same scenario, think of a time when you are stressed or in distress and think about the pros and cons of being kind/compassionate towards yourself at this time:

Advantages of being kind to self	Disadvantages at time of being kind

Try to think of what a kinder, wiser person might say to you in these circumstances. If it was someone else what might you say to them.

FIGURE 9.5 *Self-acceptance worksheet*

A copy of this figure is available to download from https://study.sagepub.com/laidlaw

Jennifer recovered her equilibrium quite quickly, and this was seen as a positive development. Jennifer reduced her self-criticism, and adopted compassionate self-acceptance, by focusing on using self-helpful statements that encouraged using her own resources to calm herself when in crisis. She was able to do this in a number of challenging situations, and she developed a sense of increasing strength from her strategies of self-soothing. An example from later on in therapy was when she bought a new car. Shortly after, it needed to be taken back to the garage for a safety-recall check. She drove to the garage herself and didn't ask anyone to sit with her in the car even though she was driving to a different garage from the one where she bought her car. She was able to see the achievement by saying: 'Proud of myself over how I have coped with it all.'

Self-compassion is an outcome of developing wisdom. Using past experiences by understanding that criticism does not help in a crisis but merely adds fuel to the fire is a very good outcome that may inoculate clients from unnecessary distress. At the end of therapy Jennifer was able to state that one of the things she had learned was that 'I could use the problems which I have experienced through my life to help me deal with stressful periods which may occur in the present or future.' Shortly after discharge Jennifer was able to go on holiday abroad for the first time in a number of years when she visited friends in Belgium.

Summary

This chapter has introduced some new techniques to consider when working with older people, and for those whose problems have longevity attached to them. The importance of understanding an individual's inner experience and belief level is also central to the ideas presented here. It is considered important that the stereotypical and biased beliefs that individuals endorse when depressed or anxious can present many challenges for symptom reduction, but these can be overcome by introducing a frame of reference of resilience and an approach based on unconditional self-acceptance. It is anticipated that wisdom may function as a vehicle for change in CBT and provide a conceptual level for process thinking about modifications to CBT with older people.

Further Reading

The following sources provide more in-depth coverage of topics raised in this chapter.

Baltes, P. B. & Smith, J. (2008). The fascination of wisdom: its nature, ontogeny, and function. *Perspectives on Psychological Science, 3*, 56–64

Bernard, M. E. (Ed.). (2013). *The strength of self-acceptance*. Melbourne: Springer Publications.

Germer, C. K. & Siegel, R. D. (Eds.). (2012). *Wisdom and compassion in psychotherapy: deepening mindfulness in clinical practice*. New York: Guilford Press.

Ten

Chronicity and Comorbidity

Learning Objectives
By the end of this chapter you will:

- Understand the different potential challenges of maintaining well-being with longstanding conditions
- Comprehend how to use CBT with older people with chronic comorbid conditions and apply clinical modifications as may be necessary
- Understand how to augment CBT for use with physical conditions using a model of ageing to optimise functioning
- Know how to approach long-term cases and treatment resistant cases using CBT, by thinking in terms of 'packages of care'

Introduction

Sooner or later when working with older people you are going to be confronted with two issues: comorbidity and chronicity. Due to improved medical procedures, people increasingly survive after strokes, heart attacks, etc., with many older people also developing non-communicable diseases.

Using standard CBT with these clients requires careful thought, as treatment may be longer and conceptualisation may be more challenging. It is important to remember when working with this client group that the experience of a physical illness is also psychological (IAPT, 2008). Therefore, it is the meaning that clients attach to their experience, informed by their health belief models, that determines the impact on a client's well-being. Conditions more common in older people are stroke, COPD, Parkinson's disease and dementia.

Complications and Comorbidity

Older people who seek out psychological help in primary care settings often have to discuss this with healthcare professionals with a lack of training in geriatric care.

Medical illnesses complicate the recognition and treatment of depression and anxiety (Krishnan et al., 2002), so older people may not receive psychological interventions as problems can seem 'understandable' and linked to ageing. Unutzer et al. (1999: 235) talk of primary care providers having a fear of opening up a 'Pandora's box' of issues when enquiring about mental health and fearing issues may come up that are difficult to contain and manage. Thus, older people may face a number of barriers in accessing psychological treatment.

Living with a limiting long-term condition may be a difficult transition for the client to navigate. You may wish to appraise yourself of a number of elements as you commence therapy:

- *Psychoeducation* about anxiety and depression. *Affective disturbance* may complicate treatment as the negativity of thinking evident in depression may leave people pessimistic about achieving rehabilitation goals, likewise anxiety about possibility of harm from engaging in activity may impede the progress clients can make.
- *Collaborative empiricism* is essential during the early phase of treatment in order to collaboratively test out the limits of what a client can realistically manage, as their sense of their abilities may be negatively influenced by anxiety and depression symptoms. Clients can become passive and hopeless, i.e. 'I am no longer able to do anything on my own,' with progress towards treatment goals compromised.
- *Problem solving* is a very useful means of brainstorming client's ideas about pragmatic ways of living well with disabilities (it indirectly encourages personal agency on a number of levels). Problem solving can present new ideas and strategies to a client and encourages them to challenge their (often mood state-dependent) thinking.
- Understanding the *nature and quality of supports* available to the person is important, as is the pre-morbid nature of the primary caregiving relationship. Look out for risk-aversive behaviours in clients and their carers that may result in passivity and dependence, i.e. 'I may injure myself if I am not careful.' Excess disability may become a significant barrier to good treatment outcome.
- Supporting *adjustment to the new reality* of life while striving towards a realistic appraisal of the impact of the condition and achievement of the highest possible level of functioning.
- It is helpful to examine clients' *mental models* and *historical experience of illness*. Very often clients will reference their understanding of illness in terms of the experience of family members. An 'n' of one rule is overgeneralised and biased, does not promote a positive sense of well-being and engenders fear for the future. Clients who know of someone who has experienced their current illness often assume their circumstances will follow the same course. For example, Peter was diagnosed with Parkinson's disease and his best friend had previously died from end-stage Parkinson's disease. This is traumatic to witness, but this experience he related to himself was unhelpful and unrealistic as the course of Parkinson's disease, as with many conditions, can be very variable (see www.nhs.uk/Conditions/Parkinsons-disease/Pages/Symptoms.aspx). Thus, therapists need to examine the client's 'experience' with the illness they are living with.

Applying CBT with Older People in the Context of Chronicity and Complexity

In a classic text, Rybarczyk et al. (1992) outline five elements that therapists need to appraise themselves of when working with comorbidity in depression and anxiety disorders: (1) practical barriers to participation in therapy; (2) accepting depression as a separate but reversible problem distinct from their ongoing physical problems; (3) identifying and limiting excess disability; (4) recognising and limiting losses of roles and autonomy; and (5) challenging self-perception of oneself as a burden to others. The structure of Rybarczyk et al. (1992) is adopted in the following sections as a reference point for therapists working with older people using CBT.

Overcoming Practical Barriers to Attending for CBT

For many older people there can be pragmatic difficulties to participating in therapy, and resolving these may require some flexibility on the part of the therapist. The therapist can do a lot to overcome physical barriers in attending outpatient appointments. Older clients can be accommodated by having appointments in rooms on a ground-floor building and by meeting the client as they exit a patient transport service. Therapists need to be sure to factor in at least ten minutes either side of the session to assist the client accessing your office. You can also be more flexible in terms of session times and treatment length. Clients can be encouraged to enlist the participation of friends or family in getting themselves to the session. It is not uncommon for clients to prefer their partner to attend their sessions with you.

Mrs Gray (see also Chapter 7) walks with two sticks and has arthritis in her wrists but drives herself (modified vehicle) to her appointments with you. As Mrs Gray can sometimes struggle with getting ready for her appointment, the therapist negotiated an 'approximate' time for appointments so she did not need to leave her house too early. At issue here is the stress older clients experience if they arrive late for their appointments. In this case it is important for the therapist to be very disciplined about being in the reception area to meet Mrs Gray in order to assist her in walking to the therapist's office.

Sometimes this kind of flexibility means that treatment length becomes prolonged because of treatment for chronic health conditions. For example, Mrs Cameron (aged 78) was initially referred for treatment for a longstanding anxiety disorder. Using graded exposure she made good progress in confronting agoraphobic symptoms (eventually she sent her therapist a postcard from South Africa, even though at the start of treatment she was unable to manage prolonged travel on buses). Over the course of therapy treatment, Mrs Cameron required two hip operations. Deciding on whether to undergo surgery was a source of considerable anxiety for her and temporarily became a focus for the sessions. Equal time was devoted to discussions about pros and cons of undergoing an operation (and tackling avoidance about finding out factual information from her doctors) and tackling her agoraphobia symptoms. The client gained great confidence in using psychological strategies to manage anxiety using graded hierarchies and graded exposure, and generalised these skills to other challenges in her life.

Depression is a Separate but Reversible Problem

Some clients find it difficult to accept depression as a separate but reversible problem distinct from their ongoing physical problems. For example, Michael has been diagnosed with prostate cancer and is undergoing treatment that leaves him tired and emotionally drained. He finds it hard to separate his depression symptoms from his physical symptoms, and at times fails to recognise that a lot of problems can be resolved by the way he thinks about the situation. Michael loses patience with himself because he used to be a very energetic and positive person. He feels his cancer has robbed him of his identity: 'I am overwhelmed by it all . . . I have no strength and stamina and I just feel swept along by an alien occupation of my body and soul as I watch from afar.'

Michael has also developed some memory difficulties that he finds frustrating: 'These petty things [forgetting] make me surge with anger [at myself] and it colours the rest of my day.' The therapist needs to help Michael to recognise that depression is as big a problem for him as is his memory and physical problems. This client has what Rybarczyk et al. (1992: 131) refer to as a belief that 'illness equals inevitable misery'. The therapist encourages Michael to review previous times in his life when he overcame challenging situations (Rybarczyk et al., 1992), and he is encouraged to keep diaries of times when he has made mistakes and to use cognitive distancing (e.g. 'if this had happened to a very close friend what would you say or do?') as a way of overcoming his frustration. Asked what he would say or do if he was aware of someone else becoming distressed in similar circumstances, he stated that 'If it was someone else I would have responded to his state, to his distress [and worked to reduce it].' Finally, Michael was coached in developing compassionate self-acceptance for his current difficulties in a way that accepts the reality of his situation without becoming passive and hopeless (see Laidlaw, 2013a).

Identifying and Limiting Excess Disability

Excess disability is where a client appears more impaired or disabled than one might expect for their stage of illness or severity of impairment. This can lead to people becoming less active and more dependent. Unfortunately, carers and healthcare workers can inadvertently reinforce cognitive and behavioural responses:

> A vicious cycle is created when the inactivity is followed by deconditioning which, in turn, leads to further restriction of activity . . . On the cognitive side, there are a number of distortions and false beliefs that impede the patient from being active. (Rybarczyk et al., 1992: 131)

Excess disability is also a risk when an older client misattributes problems with health as an inevitable consequence of age. Left unchecked this cognitive error can magnify and complicate things for older people, resulting in unhelpful safety behaviours. For example, Arthur is a keen cyclist who regularly cycles with a group of friends. Out of the blue, after a cycling trip he experienced some 'strange sensations' in his legs. Presumably due to being 81 years of age, he was advised by family friends to take it easy and he stopped cycling. His family doctor advised he engage in moderate exercise, but as Arthur experienced sensations after exercising he decided he'd 'better not take the risk of making this thing worse', and became very inactive. This had the impact of isolating Arthur from his friends and disconnecting himself from pleasant events, so he quickly became quite dejected.

There were very clear indications of safety behaviour in how Arthur responded to the sensations in his legs, and as these maintained anxiety symptoms (Salkovskis et al., 1999) he became beset with worries about the future and he started to become hyper-vigilant for further signs of deterioration in his health. After a number of investigations no identifiable cause was found. Arthur concluded that 'So far no one had come up with any ideas what could be causing my legs not to function properly.' A negative anxious cycle of thoughts plagued Arthur as follows: 'These damn legs are no better, may even be slightly worse,' 'Where is this all going to lead to?' 'I try not to think about it, but when am I going to feel better?' At its conclusion, Arthur catastrophises about the consequences of his medically unexplained symptoms: 'I might have to get out of this house sooner than I want. I will end up in a wheelchair.'

Arthur was helped to counteract his fears by focusing on facts and looking at evidence for his belief that he would become disabled. As it took time for investigations to conclude and for second opinions to be exhausted, he was able to look at predictions he had made months previously and see that they had served to heighten anxiety but did turn out to be accurate. He was also helped by being encouraged to increase his walking and to use cognitive strategies to challenge his fears. He was also encouraged to utilise distraction techniques when waiting for a diagnosis, and as a keen painter he found that this worked to take his mind off his fears: 'If I'm having a bad day, I realise the best thing is to occupy your mind, like looking for a sketch [to paint].'

Limiting Loss of Roles and Autonomy

Loss is a part of life and of ageing, but limiting the loss of valued roles and goals and maintaining autonomy is an important issue for older people. There are also bereavements or changes in physical health status for therapists to contend with. Laidlaw et al. (2003) and Laidlaw (2008b) provide examples of augmenting CBT using a model of successful ageing developed by Baltes and colleagues (Baltes & Smith, 2003; Freund & Baltes 1998) called SOC (selective optimisation with compensation). SOC is a problem-focused orientation consistent with the empowering agenda of CBT. SOC is the means by which an individual purposefully allocates his resources to produce maximal gains in a valued area. Selection implies clients may need to elect to focus on some goals over others, with compensation implying a need to change the means by which goals are achieved (Freund, 2008). Optimisation implies that when a new strategy is employed, the client needs to practice this in advance of achieving valued roles and goals. As such, SOC is an active adjustment to age-related challenges to well-being, with a shift to compensation from optimisation over the lifespan (Freund, 2008). SOC can be used in CBT when older people have realistic challenges facing them that require adjustment and adaptation. SOC reminds us that older people are resilient, and rather than responding to loss of function by giving up goals they actively seek alternative ways of achieving them. Rozario et al. (2011) illustrate how people use SOC to overcome challenges associated with chronic illnesses.

The principles of SOC are illustrated by Baltes's example of how the great concert pianist, Arthur Rubinstein, managed to successfully perform concerts late into life. When asked for the secrets of his success, Rubinstein mentioned three strategies. First, he reduced the size of his repertoire (an example of selection), and second, he practiced the restricted repertoire more intensely so there were less cognitive demands placed upon him to achieve his goal (an example of optimisation). Finally, Rubinstein created the illusion of playing fast by purposefully slowing down immediately prior to playing the faster segments of his repertoire, thereby giving his audience the impression of greater dexterity than was actually the case (an example of compensation). The orchestration of the three elements of SOC enables an individual to function at the most optimal level despite the existence of age-related challenges.

Challenging the Self-Perception of Oneself As a Burden

This is a very challenging issue to deal with in therapy, and one that may be commonly observed in people with dementia. People are partly concerned about the loss of their own independence, but they can also be distressed by the thought that family members (sons, daughters, spouses) are going to become 'encumbered' by caring for them. Often spouses and other family members want to care through a process of reciprocity, and caring can provide meaning for others as they adjust to the new challenges that the future brings. Therapists may wish to ask the person what they would expect of themselves if the places were reversed. If their spouse were the one that was facing the same problems they themselves are now facing, what would they do? If they would willingly care, then you can explore using Socratic questions how it is they are being a burden.

Similarly, when people develop physical limitations they are prone to dichotomous cognitive biases, black-and-white thinking about being useful within the family. A clear example of this is, once again, Mrs Gray. She was physically frail and unable to completely dress herself, and she felt redundant in her family believing that if she died no one would miss her. All her life she had been the strong one in the family and the person everyone looked towards to solve problems. She had equated physical strength with competence. However, she had forgotten that mostly people turned to her for her intelligence and sensible solutions to her problems. Her daughters still turned to her for advice, and although she was more dependent on her children for visiting places and shopping there was reciprocity of care. Often a sense of burden is an indication of a rigid thinking error, and can be challenged using standard cognitive techniques in CBT. Readers interested in this concept may find the CBT case study by Richardson and Marshall (2012) useful.

A Brief Introduction to Depression and Anxiety in Stroke and Parkinson's Disease

A common challenge that psychotherapists face when working with comorbidity in depression and anxiety disorders is becoming familiar with different healthcare professions, and becoming knowledgeable about symptom profiles and the consequences of neurological conditions. Readers may wish to consult simple guides produced by charities (see www.parkinsons.org.uk/sites/default/files/publications/ download/english/l001_introtoparkinsons.pdf and www.stroke.org.uk/information/resource-library). These provide succinct guides to the challenges your clients may experience and are likely to have been read by your clients, so it is useful for you to know what information they have about their condition. Diagnosis of a neurological condition like Parkinson's disease may involve a prolonged experience with carers, while the individual themselves experience fragmented care and poor information (NAO, 2011).

A Life Worth Living After a Stroke?

Stroke is one of the major causes of disability, and rates of depression and anxiety are higher than the average for community-dwelling older people. Overall, 33 per cent of people who experience a stroke will develop depression (Hackett et al., 2005). For psychologists working with people with strokes, it is important to understand the psychological impact of such a sudden, profound and catastrophic change to a person's life and future. Interested readers may wish to consult the CBT framework for post-stroke depression and anxiety (Broomfield et al., 2011).

Stroke Onset is Psychologically Challenging

A stroke often happens without warning, and is life threatening in many cases, so it can be very frightening and traumatic for the individual and their loved ones. With no warning there is simply no time to prepare for an event that changes a person's life forever. Thus, therapists need to ask about the client's experience of a stroke and the personal consequences of this. Often the client or family member may become fearful that another event will strike without warning. The therapist needs to be attentive to the development of safety behaviours that a client may engage in following such a profoundly important life event.

Evidence-Based CBT for Comorbid Physical Illness

Post-Stroke Depression

For post-stroke depression (PSD), it can be said that CBT *should* work in reducing post-stroke morbidity, rather than it *does* work. Unfortunately, two separate RCTs evaluating non-modified CBT have produced disappointing results. Studies that have evaluated CBT have done so from a non-augmented perspective, and this may ignore the context in which a person experiences negative cognitions about stroke and stroke recovery. Nevertheless, there are good grounds for recommending CBT for PSD and anxiety, as it empowers individuals during their rehabilitation from stroke and equips clients with problem-oriented strategies that can enhance mood (Broomfield et al., 2011).

One of the most challenging issues when working with clients with PSD is that they often want to make a 100 per cent recovery and anything less is seen as insufficient. This can lead to a significant cognitive error, termed a baseline distortion

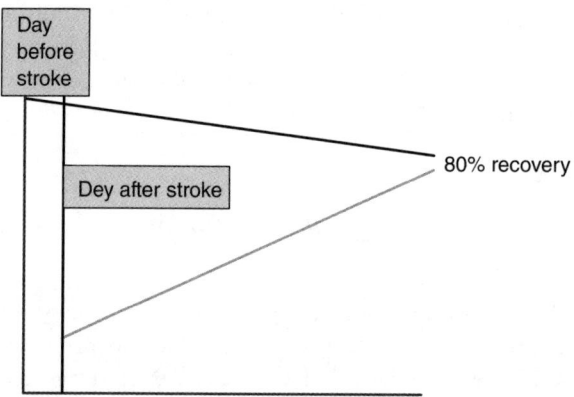

It's how you look at the evidence. It's in the eye of the beholder. What seems a fairer comparison to you?

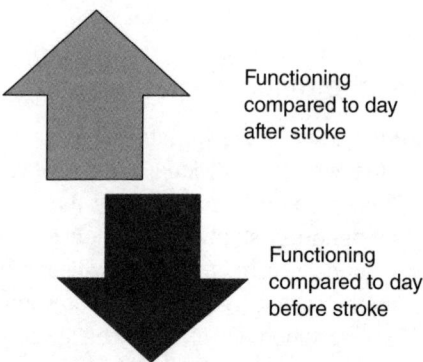

FIGURE 10.1 *Stroke baseline distortion worksheet*

(Laidlaw, 2008b). This is where a person with PSD negatively appraises progress made in post-stroke recovery as they compare their current functioning with that of their functioning *prior* to a stroke. This is obviously a false comparison to make, as the states of living with a stroke are qualitatively different from that of not living with a stroke. There is a negative filter towards negative construal, when in fact a more logical comparison is between functioning currently and function immediately after the stroke occurred. A useful diagram is shown in Figure 10.1 to illustrate this point. With the baseline set appropriately, a client can appreciate the progress that is being made. It is recommended that this graph is used early on in therapy as a good way to socialise clients to the cognitive model.

Depression in Parkinson's Disease

Parkinson's disease affects approximately 120,000 people in the UK with approximately 10,000 new cases every year. Parkinson's disease is characterised by bradykinesia (slowness of movement), tremor at rest, rigidity, balance problems and abnormality of gait. These motor symptoms of Parkinson's disease interfere with everyday tasks that people take for granted, such as buttoning one's shirt. Non-motor symptoms such as depression and anxiety may affect up to 40 per cent of people with Parkinson's disease and are often under-recognised, not least because an accurate diagnosis of depression in Parkinson's disease is complicated because of the overlap between neurological and psychological symptoms.

The evidence for CBT for depression in Parkinson's disease is still developing (Charidimou et al., 2011). Currently treatment outcome of medication for depression in Parkinson's disease remains at best inconclusive (Troeung et al., 2013). A recent case study by Richardson and Marshall (2012) has demonstrated that CBT has utility for treating depression even in more advanced stages of Parkinson's disease. Dobkin et al. (2011) produced a large robust evaluation of CBT for depression in Parkinson's disease, with participants randomly allocated to two treatment groups: CBT plus clinical management (CBT+CM) versus clinical management alone (CMA). More than half (56 per cent) in the CBT+CM group, compared to less than one in ten (8 per cent) in the CMA group, met predefined criteria as treatment responders at end of treatment. Until this point the psychological treatment literature was based around open trials and small case study series. In a recent review of CBT for depression in Parkinson's disease, Charidimou et al. (2011: 7) conclude that:

> If shown to be effective in large RCTs, CBT could potentially provide a better possible nonpharmacologic treating option for clinicians for the treatment of depression in PD [Parkinson's disease], either when pharmacotherapy fails, in combination or as an alternative to pharmacological treatment of dPD [depression in Parkinson's disease].

CBT can be a good fit for depression in Parkinson's disease, as the emphasis is on developing strategies and skills to compensate for problems that often arise from erroneous appraisals of situations during a depressive episode (Laidlaw, 2008c). Sessions focus upon appraisals clients make with regard to their experience of life after diagnosis. A useful strategy at this point is to introduce a phase model of grief (i.e. Worden (2009) defined stages of mourning, bargaining and denial, anger, acceptance and moving on) to help participants come to terms with Parkinson's disease and focus more explicitly upon what aspects of life they appraise to be most keenly felt in terms of loss post-diagnosis. Although people living with Parkinson's disease often have to deal with realistic challenges, individuals nevertheless often endorse unhelpful or erroneous cognitions about these challenges. It is important that therapists assist the client in dealing with current problems in the here and now, while being aware that clients have fears about their anticipated future with Parkinson's disease. Therapists can help clients recognise and manage 'fortune telling' errors.

Managing Comorbidity in CBT: An Integrative Conceptualisation

When working with clients with physical comorbid conditions in depression and anxiety, there can be multiple causal and contributory factors to take account of, and very rarely will these be entirely psychological. Kinderman and Tai (2007) have developed a useful conceptualisation framework that works well in understanding the impact of the confluence of physical and psychological phenomena at the level of the experience of the individual. In this model, Kinderman and Tai (2007: 2) propose that 'Biological and environmental factors, together with a person's personal experiences, lead to mental

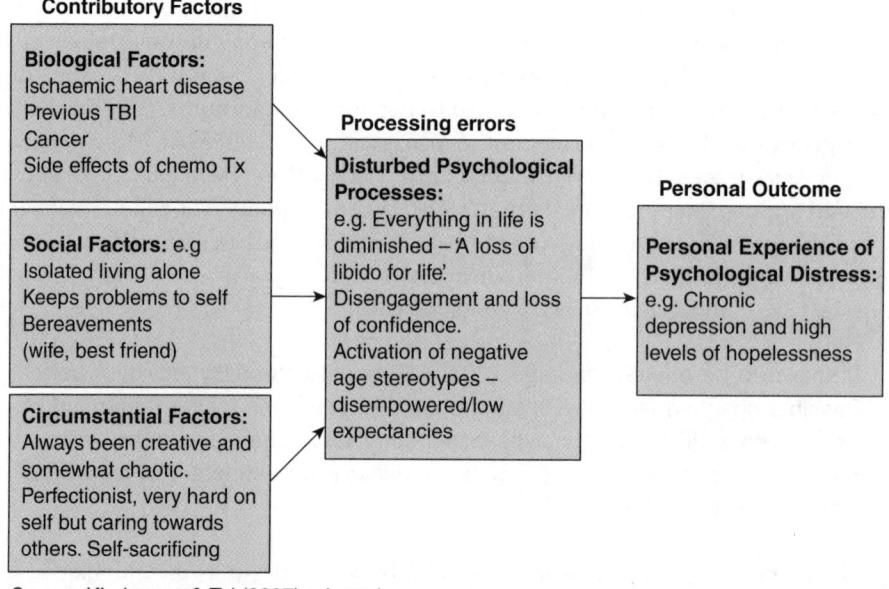

Source: Kinderman & Tai (2007) adapted

FIGURE 10.2 *Conceptualising CBT interventions via psychological processes*

disorder through their conjoint effects on these psychological processes.' The elegant simplicity of this model makes it easy to describe to clients and provides a way of making sense of their experiences that acknowledges the realistic challenges of living with physical illness and maintaining an equilibrium in emotional well-being. An example of this model is illustrated in Figure 10.2, with reference to Michael who has cancer and depression. In this model, how an individual makes sense of their experiences can be useful in normalising an individual's distress. For Michael this model has a powerful explanatory role in how it is that they experience their illness in the way they do, and how they respond in a way that promotes greater distress. The disturbed psychological processes suggest the way forward for interventions with Michael.

Managing Chronicity: CBT for Longer-Term Complex Cases

Often when working with older people there are clients who are referred for psychological therapy with longstanding mental health challenges stretching over decades. These clients can have a long history of contact with psychiatric services, and are often socialised into expecting very little in the way of beneficial treatment outcome. These clients can be challenging to work with, as they often have very poor quality of life, are sometimes 'blamed' by healthcare professionals for the ongoing nature of their difficulties, and are frequently prescribed medications that don't resolve the nature of the client's distress (McCullough, 2012). Therapists can be concerned about taking these clients on, so in many ways these clients are exceptionally vulnerable and are often seen as challenging for other colleagues to manage, and can be referred even when previous referrals have mainly contained, rather than addressed, distress. In these circumstances it may make sense to think in terms of 'packages of treatment'. It seems imprudent to expect a 'cure' from a 16–20 session treatment if someone has been in contact with psychiatric services for more than 16–20 years. It can be demoralising to both the therapist and the client if realistic expectations for treatment gains are not explicitly outlined at the start of treatment.

An example of a 'packages of treatment' approach in CBT with older people is outlined by work with Mrs Lenahan. This client had been seen by three different psychological therapists over the last four years and had a very large case file, with multiple healthcare professionals involved in her care over the last decade. She had been seen by each therapist for at least one year and had always returned to therapy with the same issues unresolved. Discharge had always been arrived at in the same way. She and the therapist 'took a break' from ongoing contact, so Mrs Lenahan was being socialised into expecting an unresolved outcome for psychological therapy. When Mrs Lenahan was referred again to the service, the therapist discussed what she had gained from her previous treatment. She found the accepting stance of therapists to be important to her, but she did not enjoy having to do homework tasks as she really wanted someone to be there for her when life became difficult. The therapist outlined a standard CBT approach and collaboratively drew up a problem list highlighting homework as an essential component of treatment. Top of Mrs Lenahan's problem list was communication problems with her eldest son. Mrs Lenahan's son had a number of childhood illnesses that meant he was hospitalised, and as a result Mrs Lenahan believed she hadn't bonded with him. This was a powerful explanatory construct that she came back to time and again in her description of the nature of her relationship difficulties. It did not, however, point to any here-and-now interventions that she could implement, and did not help improve her relationship. She also stated that her husband was unsupportive and uncommunicative, which she explained as 'what men are like'. She saw herself in very negative terms, which again contributed to a general sense of lack of personal agency. The therapist and Mrs Lenahan agreed to focus on improving communication as the sole focus for this package of care. The idea stuck, and the therapist and client worked towards a simple goal and remained focused on this despite other problems occasionally intruding. Nevertheless, the focus was helpful for Mrs Lenahan, and as a by-product the resolution of some communication difficulties with her son also challenged her personal attributions about her ability to bring about positive change in her personal circumstances. As agreed, Mrs Lenahan was discharged from therapy. This was the first time in many years that Mrs Lenahan had been discharged in this way. Packages of care allow the therapist and client to achieve focus, and allow the therapist to become active and directive in treatment without feeling they are non-responsive to chaotic or challenging issues that may also threaten outcome towards agreed goals.

Summary and Conclusions

Working with clients with chronic and comorbid conditions can be challenging and may even be dispiriting for therapists and their clients. Although it is unintentional, an acute model of CBT may be applied that is less likely to be effective. If there are complicating comorbid issues a standard CBT formulation may not be entirely successful, and goals for treatment outcome in the light of chronicity stretching back decades need careful negotiation and consideration.

Learning Log: Reflection and Review

- Can you think of a client that you learned a lot from? What outcome did you achieve together and how does this compare with the evidence base for this presentation or client group?
- Working with comorbid conditions often means understanding more about common age-related neurological conditions such as stroke and Parkinson's disease. Perhaps a plan for CPD could include attending seminars on these conditions?
- Often charities and support groups for people with neurological conditions arrange one-day local conferences that are an excellent way to understand the personal impact of chronic conditions.
- Could you justify your interventions and outcome for more complex cases based on outcome? Consider what additional gains, other than symptom reduction, may have been achieved over the course of treatment (e.g. less attendance at A&E, less GP appointments, etc.).

Further Reading

The following sources provide more in-depth coverage of topics raised in this chapter.

NICE (2009). *Depression in adults with a chronic physical health problem: treatment and management*. NICE Clinical Guideline 91. Available at: www.nice.org. uk/nicemedia/live/12327/45909/45909.pdf

Safren, S., Gonzalez, J., & Soroudi, N. (2008). *Coping with chronic illness: a cognitive-behavioral approach for adherence and depression therapist guide (treatments that work)*. New York: Oxford University Press.

White, C. A. (2001). *Cognitive behaviour therapy for chronic medical problems: a guide to assessment and treatment in practice*. Chichester: John Wiley & Sons.

Eleven

CBT for People with Dementia and Their Carers

Learning Objectives

By the end of this chapter you will:

- Know about dementia prevalence and types and how this may impact upon therapy process
- Recognise the efficacy of CBT for people with depression and/or anxiety in dementia
- Appreciate the efficacy of CBT for dementia caregivers
- Understand how to transform theory into practice in order to work with people with dementia and their caregivers using CBT principles and techniques
- Be able to apply some standard CBT techniques in novel ways with caregivers

Introduction

CBT is likely to be a good fit for people with depression or anxiety in dementia, as the non-stigmatising, collaborative and structured nature of this approach is likely to match the needs of clients, empowering them to find ways to compensate for memory or other cognitive impairments in order to function optimally. An evidence-based psychological approach for depression and anxiety in dementia is particularly necessary when one realises that inconsistent evidence exists for the efficacy of pharmacotherapy for people with dementia (Enache et al., 2011). CBT is also consistent with an ethical approach to dementia, promoting autonomy, solidarity and inclusion (Nuffield Council on Bioethics, 2009). The UK government (see House of Lords, 2013) expects 80 per cent more people with dementia over the age of 65 in 2030 compared to 2010. As people with dementia are likely to be identified earlier and diagnosed more accurately, potentially many more people will be faced with a life-changing diagnosis and may experience considerable distress about what the future might hold for them and their family. Dementia care is therefore likely to be an issue that therapists are increasingly familiar with.

Introduction to Dementia

Around 820,000 people live with dementia in the UK, with the annual cost estimated at around £23 billion – more than heart disease and cancer care combined (Luengo-Fernandez et al., 2010). Most care for people with dementia is provided within the family (WHO, 2012). Carers require considerable support in order to remain in their role looking after loved ones. The World Health Organization (WHO, 2012) estimates that there are currently 36 million people living with dementia globally, and that this will double every twenty years, reaching 66 million in 2030 and increasing to 115 million by 2050. Both England and Scotland have national dementia programmes produced in 2009 and 2010 respectively (for England's approach, see www.dh.gov.uk/prod_consum_dh/groups/dh_digitalassets/@dh/@en/documents/digitalasset/dh_094051.pdf and for Scotland's approach see www.scotland.gov.uk/Resource/Doc/324377/0104420.pdf).

Dementia is a global public health and social care priority (WHO, 2012). However, dementia is *not* an inevitable outcome of old age. Consistent with most dementias, Alzheimer's disease is more common in older people, with prevalence increasing with age and doubling every five years for men and women. While the main risk factor for developing dementia is age (Alzheimer's Association, 2011), the therapist needs to remember that this does not mean that if a person lives long enough they will definitely get dementia. The *Dementia 2010* report (Luengo-Fernandez et al., 2010) notes that between the ages of 95 and 99 years, 32 per cent of men and 36 per cent of women have dementia. The full figures are detailed in Table 11.1.

Dementia is an Umbrella Term

Dementia is an umbrella term for a progressive brain condition describing a cluster of symptoms such as problems with planning, thinking and reasoning, memory,

TABLE 11.1   *Prevalence rates for dementia in the UK (males and females)*

Age range	Prevalence (males) %	Prevalence (females) %
60–64	1.58	0.47
65–69	2.17	1.10
70–74	4.61	3.86
75–79	5.04	6.67
80–84	12.12	13.50
85–89	18.45	22.76
90–94	32.10	32.25
95–99	31.58	36.00

Source: Dementia 2010: Luengo-Fernandez, Leal, Gray, 2010

behaviour, personality change and the ability to perform everyday functions that we all take for granted, such as communicating and dressing. Often people with dementia develop physical problems, and in time can become quite dependent upon other people and health and social services for care (Luengo-Fernandez et al., 2010; WHO, 2012). Dementia progressively impacts upon an individual's ability to moderate environments, both internally and externally. As dementia progresses, the ability of a person to adapt to stress levels may become impaired, and therefore anxiety and depression can become an additional challenge for people to overcome.

There are many different types of dementia and many different causes, with Alzheimer's disease being the most common type (60 per cent of people with dementia are diagnosed with this condition). This is followed by vascular dementia (previously known as multi-infarct dementia) and Lewy body dementia, accounting for about 15–20 per cent of all cases (Luengo-Fernandez et al., 2010). Different dementias (Alzheimer's, vascular, Lewy body, frontotemporal, etc.) may have different neuropsychological profiles (Aarsland et al., 2001; Bondi et al., 2009; Caputo et al., 2008; Palmqvist et al., 2009).

It may be useful to take account of potential differences when working with people with different dementias. However, this can be a very complex and challenging area for practitioners without an understanding of neuropsychology. Dementias can be classified as cortical or subcortical, for example (Fletcher et al., 2007). Dementia with Lewy bodies (DLB) is a subcortical dementia, whereas Alzheimer's disease is a cortical dementia (Bondi et al., 2009), although there is overlap in symptoms between the two conditions as DLB may also have some cortical dysfunction and is often misdiagnosed as Alzheimer's disease (Palmqvist et al., 2009). A common feature in DLB is cognitive fluctuation, but this is also present to a lesser extent in people with Alzheimer's disease, and the accurate assessment of cognitive fluctuation remains elusive (Lee et al., 2012).

> Dementia can be thought of as a journey, and the active-directive non-stigmatising problem-oriented approach adopted in CBT may be very useful in navigating this journey more successfully. Goals for treatment may be different – for example, it may be maintaining function and reducing risk rather than seeking cure.

The profile of different dementias is highly complex and is beyond the scope of this book. Therapists inexperienced in understanding neuropsychological profiles in dementia may wish to consult clinical neuropsychologists prior to embarking upon CBT treatment. When working with people with dementia it is especially important to take a comprehensive history and to recruit a carer to help with monitoring the current nature of the difficulties experienced by the person with dementia. A number of studies reporting on the use of cognitive and behavioural therapies with older people with dementia have reported on the use of confederate family members in treatments (Kiosses et al., 2011; Paukert et al., 2010).

Preparing to Work with People with Dementia: Evidence Base

Depression in dementia is complex to treat with evidence for antidepressants currently inconclusive (Enache et al., 2011; Orgeta et al., 2014). Thus, there is a need to consider whether psychological therapy may have a role to play in treatment options for people with dementia and their carers. Diagnosing anxiety and depression in dementia is a complex issue and beyond the scope of this chapter, but if in doubt check diagnostic status with colleagues making referrals for treatment.

> To paraphrase Tom Kitwood's more positivist person-centred approach, one ought to facilitate the following in people living with dementia: a sense of personal worth, a sense of agency, social confidence, and hope (Kitwood, 1997) CBT shares these values and philosophical position.

When working with people with anxiety and depression in dementia, it is currently unclear at which point CBT interventions will become ineffective due to cognitive decline, and therefore the therapist may wish to track this using behavioural experiments as a guide. Although the goals of treatment may be different, such as optimising functioning or managing uncertainty, the symptom-focused aspect of CBT remains the same.

Evidence for the efficacy of CBT in anxiety and depression in dementia comes mainly from a range of small intriguing clinical trials and case studies. Mohlman and Gorman (2005) note that treatment outcome for CBT for anxiety disorder can be compromised when clients have executive dysfunction (i.e. specific cognitive deficits in planning, organising and reasoning abilities). If attention training and enhanced self-monitoring in therapy are used to augment CBT, deficits can be overcome and enhanced treatment outcome achieved (Mohlman & Gorman, 2005). The evidence base for CBT interventions for people with anxiety or depression in dementia is summarised in Table 11.2.

Orgeta et al. (2014) reviewed evidence for psychological interventions for people with anxiety and depression in mild dementia, and while six RCTs were identified, all but one were considered at high risk for bias due to methodological aspects (randomisation, blinding, etc.). Psychological interventions have the potential to reduce depression and anxiety (when using clinician reports) and to improve psychological well-being in people with dementia.

Preparing to Work with People with Dementia: Diagnosis Sharing

The majority of people with dementia (92 per cent) wish to be told of their diagnosis of dementia, although data suggest the term Alzheimer's disease has more negative

TABLE 11.2 *Evidence for CBT for people with dementia*

Author (s)	Primary focus	Design	Sample size	Outcome
Teri, 1994	Depression	Open trial	22 BT and 19 control (this is the intern report for Teri et al., 1997).	Treatment took place over 9 weekly sessions of behavioural therapy, including CG in the intervention. 68 per cent of CG clinically depressed at start. 20/22 PwD improved and CGs also shown improvement. No change evident in W/L control group.
Teri et al., 1997	Depression	Open trial	72 dyads: BT-PE, BT-PS, TAU and W/L. CGs involved actively.	Both active treatments more effective in reducing depression than TAU or W/L. 60 per cent of participants in active BT conditions improved and 70 per cent in TAU and W/L show no improvement. CGs depression improved significantly and changes in carers and PwD maintained at 6-month follow-up.
Koder, 1998	Anxiety	Single cases	2	Two single cases of 82-year-old males with depression and anxiety. Treatment involved carers, and positive effects were reported in both cases. Treatment was structured and time-limited in both cases.
Scholey & Woods, 2003	Depression	Single cases	7	Individualised treatment protocol used without apparent difficulty. 2 out of 7 participants evidencing clinically significant improvement in mood using standardised mood scales.
Walker, 2004	Depression	Single case	1	Male living with carer, both demoralised at intake. Treatment non-responsive to ADM. Couple seen together for sixteen sessions of CBT. At end of Tx and 12-month follow-up, cognition improved (MMSE) and anxiety (GHQ 32 at b/l, 5 at follow-up) improved.
Kraus et al., 2008	Anxiety	Single cases	2	Treatment emphasises active self-monitoring by the clients (i.e. keeping a notebook handy to remember and monitor homework tasks, use of checklists to remain oriented to task and time). Emphasis on behavioural rather than cognitive change. Specific strategies used to enhance recall such as use of cues and other retrieval-based strategies.

Author (s)	Primary focus	Design	Sample size	Outcome
Kiosses et al., 2011	Depression	RCT (interim data)	15 PATH vs 15 ST	12-week home-delivered PATH (problem adaptation therapy). A behavioural problem-solving treatment was compared to 12 weeks of supportive therapy (ST) for people with depression in dementia. CG actively involved in treatment. PATH participants 51 per cent greater improvement in depression compared to ST.
Paukert et al., 2010	Anxiety	Open trial	9 intervention, 7 complete Tx	Six-month treatment with weekly session for first 12 weeks followed by telephone sessions. Carers active participants in treatment. Most participants reduced anxiety and depression, and carers concerns about PwD reduced over treatment.
Spector et al., 2013	Anxiety	RCT	25 CBT, 25 TAU	Random allocation to either CBT or treatment as usual (TAU). The CBT participants reported gains in anxiety and depression symptoms not shared by TAU participants. Gains were maintained at 6 months after follow-up, and CBT participants alone reported improvement in their relationships.

connotations (Robinson et al., 2011). Informal carers, while also being in favour of disclosure of dementia diagnosis, may be less in favour than people with dementia (Robinson et al., 2011). Thus, the therapist working with people with dementia needs to undertake a careful analysis of what information has been shared about diagnosis, and by whom and with what certainty. This is especially important as diagnosis does not take place at the same time for everyone. Neither does dementia always begin at the time of diagnosis (Scholey & Woods, 2003), with some people diagnosed earlier and others later. The person will likely have lived with dementia symptoms for some time before coming to the attention of mental health services. It is also very important when taking a history to ascertain if there is any family history of dementia, as the person may have developed expectations based on what they have witnessed family members experience. This can be a very frightening thing for a person with dementia and requires very careful handling by the therapist.

The diagnosis of dementia has implications and ramifications that go beyond the impact on the person with dementia, as family members and especially the primary caregivers will find that life and future expectations are changed following diagnosis (Nuffield Council of Bioethics, 2009).

Preparing to Work with People with Dementia: Stigmatisation

People with dementia can feel marginalised within society and may feel stigmatised (WHO, 2012), to the extent that they avoid talking about dementia for fear of losing friendships or being treated differently, and as a consequence people do not ask for help to manage dementia better as the consequences of stigma are potentially so great. Alzheimer's Disease International (ADI, 2012) carried out a global survey into stigma associated with dementia, recruiting 2,500 people with dementia and their carers (see www.alz.co.uk/research/WorldAlzheimerReport2012.pdf). A significant minority (24 per cent) conceal their diagnosis from others, 40 per cent felt they were treated differently and 59 per cent felt that they had lost contact with friends as a result of being diagnosed with dementia. For the sample as a whole, three-quarters answered yes when asked if there were negative associations of dementia in the country they lived in, with 28 per cent stating they felt marginalised.

> 'In all stages, the stigma associated with dementia also leads to a focus on the ways in which a person is impaired, rather than on his or her remaining strengths and ability to enjoy many activities and interactions with other people' (ADI, 2012: 10).

Thus, therapists working people with dementia and their carers need to consider how stigma may act as a mediator for poorer mental health. For instance, Mrs Jervis was afraid of her friends discovering her husband had Alzheimer's disease. She was embarrassed by her husband's memory failures and inability to follow conversations, so she attempted to hide his diagnosis from her friends. Of course, this proved increasingly difficult and she cut herself off from an important source of support. Following a Socratic dialogue exploring the sharing of information with her friends while maintaining her husband's dignity, she decided to 'risk' leaking the news to some close friends. The therapist used a paradoxical intention with Mrs Jervis. In order to retain control of the information about her husband's dementia she paradoxically had to give up some control of the information by sharing it, but as she was giving out the message she was in control and therefore was set to receive understanding and help from close friends. It ought to be evident to most readers that Mrs Jervis's control of information was always illusory. Nevertheless, she and her husband were helped to step back from secrecy and isolation. Once friends knew, her fears about stigmatisation were not realised. In terms of CBT it is good practice to ensure that clients write out predictions for actions in advance of taking them, and then compare the expectations with actual data.

Psychotherapy for Depression and Anxiety in Dementia

An interesting review provided by Bonder (1994) recommended that psychotherapists working with people with dementia should:

- Focus on post-diagnostic stress management
- Enhance existing and preserved coping strategies
- Affirm the person's sense of identity
- Provide individualised support
- Afford the expression of emotions
- Restore a sense of order by recognising the person's intellectual abilities

Although Bonder (1994) was not writing from a CBT-based perspective, his description is consistent with that of an approach recognising the individualised nature of the experience for the client. It is not the situation (in this case, diagnosis of dementia) that determines the impact, but the meanings ascribed to it by the individual through their idiosyncratic appraisals of the meanings this diagnosis carries for them, and its highly personalised projected ramifications for themselves and their loved ones. This standard concept in CBT translates well to people with dementia. Thus, if people are socialised into expecting that following a diagnosis with dementia they are incompetent and 'broken' they will act as such.

CBT for People with Dementia

Psychological therapists have often shied away from working with older people with dementia, as they assume that such clients will be unable to engage in the process of therapy. However, this is disempowering of individuals and is contrary to the ethos of

CBT. Many people diagnosed with dementia in the early stages will retain enough insight and capacity to engage in therapy as long as simple adjustments are made by the therapists to accommodate any mild memory or communication difficulties.

> The therapist cannot assume that a person with dementia lacks the capacity to engage, and whether this is possible can only be truly answered once a fuller assessment has been undertaken.

CBT is adapted to fit the needs of the client and not the other way round. What may be needed are more frequent summaries and a more active stance on the part of the therapist. Homework is still an important part of therapy, and behavioural experiments become even more important in understanding what a person can do.

Unless there is strong evidence that cognitive elements such as thought challenging are beyond the person's capability, the full techniques of CBT should be called upon when working with people with dementia. Remember, the person with dementia has a rich life history that they can be encouraged to draw upon to help themselves deal with the challenges of living well with dementia. Asking clients and their carers to think back to times in the past (people with dementia have a relatively better long-term memory function) when they dealt with a difficult situation and to reflect on what they learned (reflect on expectations for a good outcome, how they coped with uncertainty, etc.) may be useful for preparing the person to function more optimally with the uncertainties and challenges dementia can present to the individual and the couple.

The opinions and views of those around the older person with dementia can be important in determining how well an individual makes an adjustment to life after diagnosis. In the interests of supporting loved ones, carers sometimes inadvertently reinforce a sense of risk in the person with dementia, as there is a fear they might become disoriented when out in unfamiliar surroundings or may be at enhanced risk of embarrassment when completing everyday tasks on their own. While it is understandable that carers sometimes adopt a low-risk strategy in order to protect their loved ones, there needs to be consideration given to the impact of the loss of independence on the person with dementia and the risks associated with this in terms of their self-identity (Manthorpe & Moriarty, 2010).

For example, prior to her husband developing dementia, Mrs Lewin and her husband Anthony regularly visited a local coffee shop on the High Street. This was something the couple enjoyed doing as Mr Lewin particularly enjoyed going up to the counter and ordering. When he was diagnosed with dementia, Mrs Lewin suggested she should do the ordering now as she wanted to 'protect' her husband from the 'risk of embarrassment' in case he got confused or forgot his order. This safety–first behaviour (Manthorpe & Moriaty, 2010), done in the spirit of love and companionship, was misplaced as this had the effect of reducing Mr Lewin's confidence and increasing his sense of becoming incompetent.

Working with clients with an ongoing deteriorating condition such as dementia may be a challenging concept for some, so prior to working with your client (and their carer, as appropriate) you may wish to consider the following checklist.

Checklist for Planning to Use CBT with People with Dementia

1. Has the person been given a diagnosis, and if so by whom? Does the person know their diagnosis? Clarify the open and honest approach of CBT with clients.
2. What type of dementia has been diagnosed (this may be ascertained by talking with the referring psychiatrist or GP). Assess whether there are hallucinations or delusions experienced by the person with dementia.
3. Has a screening assessment or a comprehensive neuropsychological assessment been completed? If so, ask to see a copy of the report, or the results of the screen.
4. Does the person with dementia have a person they would identify as their primary caregiver? Would the carer(s) identify themselves as such?

   i. Sensitively assess the pre-morbid nature of their relationship before dementia was diagnosed. Importantly assess how they worked together in the past to solve problems.
   ii. Has anyone else in the family experienced dementia before. What was the nature of the relationship (e.g. mother, grandfather, etc.).
   iii. Is there a power-of-attorney arrangement in place, or planned?
   iv. Consider whether to recruit the carer as a confederate in therapy, and if so set clear ground rules in advance about confidentiality and other safeguards regarding the sharing of sensitive information.

5. Set up ground rules for how the privacy and dignity of both partners in the dyad is maintained. Make sure everything is open and transparent. Do not exclude the person with dementia. Give them time to answer questions. By modelling this approach you may help the carer to adopt a similar approach that may reduce the potential for the development of excess disability.
6. Are there identifiable behaviour or personality changes? Has anyone noticed or commented on them to the person with dementia.
7. Identify what are the main difficulties or problems experienced by the client, and what are their main concerns.

   i. Use this information to develop a problem list.
   ii. Transform this list into goals and targets for treatment.
   iii. Think about whether the aim is maintenance or enhancement of function.

8. Use a mood screen with the person. If the dementia is at a mild stage consider using the GDS and the GAI. Both have some evidence of being valid with older people with mild cognitive impairment (Boddice et al., 2008; O'Riordan et al., 1990).
9. Be positive about the possibility of change. Maintain a strong collaborative emphasis. The person with dementia still has expertise and experience that you need to tap into.
10. Don't forget to develop a conceptualisation and share this with your client and their carer. Modify and revise as necessary.

At the early post-diagnosis stage in the experience of dementia, an individual can benefit greatly from psychotherapy as they grapple with a change in their sense of self. Depressive attributions about how an individual with dementia characterises their problems may also be a useful focus for CBT interventions (Walker, 2004). Thus, if an individual attributes all memory, reasoning or communication failures to the onset of dementia symptoms this may be an overgeneralisation that ought to be tested for its veracity, as left unaddressed it is likely to be corrosive to the individual's view of self-agency and self-confidence. It may be that as an individual attempts to come to terms with failing memory they need to be reminded about the importance of challenging a view of self that is seen as impaired. Although people living with dementia have to deal with realistic challenges, they can still endorse many unhelpful or erroneous cognitions that make living with dementia much more difficult.

When working with people with dementia there may be important data to be derived from understanding how an individual reacts in response to actual or real memory failings. A disproportionate reaction can leave an individual feeling more diminished as a competent person, and this could have an adverse approach on a person's cognition, affect and behaviour.

Let's consider the following example. Michael has a mild level of memory impairment, and he becomes very agitated and distressed with what he perceives as his memory lapses.

As Figure 11.1 shows, Michael discovers that he has mislaid his bus pass when he goes to the shop to renew it. He is embarrassed at the shop and this generates a huge level of negative affect. He castigates himself over doing this and is very frustrated and upset. He says: 'That's the sort of careless thing I have begun to do,' and 'Because I have so little in my head, I'm getting more and more anxious about it [memory]. This is a feeling of entrapment. Life is defined by memory and if memory is not coherent it is very distressing.'

The real problem here isn't that Michael has mislaid his bus pass, but the affect generated when he loses things. He catastrophises that this indicates a serious memory failing and he selectively focuses on all the times he has forgotten something. It is not long

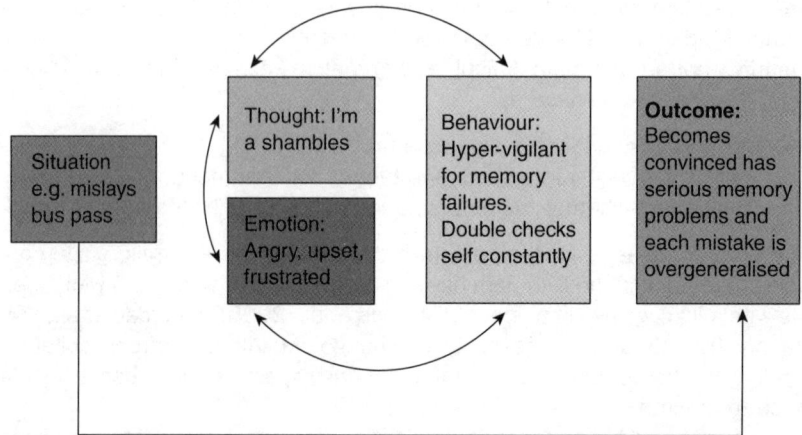

FIGURE 11.1   *Identifying negative self-defeating cycles using simple conceptualisations*

before Michael feels demoralised and hopeless. This can be understood psychologically, not only for its immediate impact but also for the long-term consequences for Michael as it increases a sense of chaos and reinforces his sense of his own incompetence. This sets up an expectancy bias, and if the therapist is not careful a vicious cycle can be set in train, as indicated in Figure 11.1, between the situation and the outcome.

The here-and-now orientation of CBT is also potentially helpful with people with dementia. Remaining in control of what is changeable is empowering and confidence-enhancing for people. The reality is that no one can foretell the future, and this remains equally true when living with dementia. Acting as if one's future is predetermined is likely to engender passivity in an individual, resulting in elevated levels of hopelessness and despair. CBT allows individuals to face their fears of an anticipated future *one day at a time.*

CBT with Caregivers

Rosalynn Carter, wife of former US President Jimmy Carter, once famously said: 'There are four kinds of people in this world: those who have been caregivers, those who currently are caregivers, those who will be caregivers, and those who will need caregivers.'

As may already be evident, CBT with people with dementia often involves working with dementia caregivers. Often when working with caregivers you will be working with the dyad (the couple), and this is equally the case when working with a person with dementia. An important consideration is the nature of the current and past relationship between the carer and the person with dementia. The experience of carers is quite different depending on whether they are spouses or adult children. Pinquart and Sorensen (2011) report that spousal caregivers use less informal support, but provide more care and experience more depressive symptoms than adult-child caregivers. As you set out to work with your client you need to explore sensitively the pre-morbid nature of the relationship between the care-provider and care-recipient. Another factor to consider is the perception that carers have about the suffering and distress experienced by their loved ones living with dementia, as this significantly contributes to caregiver suffering (Monin & Schulz, 2009). Practitioners inexperienced in working with people with dementia may wish to consult a recent guide from the Alzheimer's Society (2011).

Efficacy of CBT with Caregivers

Recently, two comprehensive reports have been published that reviewed the evidence base for caregiver interventions. Goy et al. (2010) was funded by the US Veterans

TABLE 11.3 *Brief summary of recent systematic reviews of CBT dementia caregiver interventions*

Authors	Level of analysis	Results	Conclusions
Cooke et al., 2001.	Identified types of psychosocial interventions used in CG studies. 40 papers published since 1985 met criteria for inclusion in the systematic review.	15 different interventions based on external criteria but quality was very variable. The differentiation of interventions was problematic as it mixed treatment modalities with different types of broader intervention strategies. This tends to present a confusing picture. Outcomes were classified in terms of 5 main outcomes.	'Overall, there is little evidence that interventions consistently produced benefits for caregivers in terms of improved caregiver psychological well-being or caregiver burden' (Cooke et al., 2001: 129).
Sorensen et al., 2002.	78 caregiver intervention studies covering 6 different types of interventions. Majority of studies report outcome for burden and depression.	PT and PE interventions had significant outcome on depression, burden, well-being, knowledge and care-recipient symptoms. MC interventions less effective for depression but reported improvements on burden, well-being and knowledge in caregivers.	Overall studies report small-to-moderate effects for interventions. Most consistently effective interventions are PT and PE. MC interventions had largest effect on burden, and this was larger than that achieved by PT and PE. The methodologies of studies varied as did quality. Some indication that individual interventions are more effective than group interventions.
Brodaty, 2003.	30 controlled studies of interventions with dementia caregivers. Studies included were very heterogeneous in terms of patents and caregivers.	Effect sizes were calculated to compare effectiveness of caregiver interventions, with a positive effect overall for psychosocial interventions. On average a caregiver in treatment was less depressed than 62 per cent of CGs in control conditions. Interventions that enhanced skill of PWD report better outcomes.	Modest but significant gains in psychological morbidity and in CG knowledge. Indications that CG interventions may delay institutionalisation. Short educational programmes, support groups alone and single interviews are unsuccessful interventions.

Authors	Level of analysis	Results	Conclusions
Pinquart and Sorensen, 2006.	127 studies comparing several different types of interventions with caregivers, including PE, CBT, counselling, general support, respite, etc.	CG interventions have domain-specific outcomes. Thus active PE had strongest effects (medium) on knowledge of carers, and CBT showed strongest effect on depression (large) and CG burden (medium). Structured MC interventions associated with delayed institutionalisation.	Interventions that stress active participation in CG have better long-term effects. Interventions are likely to have better outcome if they are targeted (e.g. CBT for depression). Other aspects are important in determining outcome, such as gender, age and nature of relationship of caregivers. CG interventions effective on a range of targets.
Gallagher-Thompson and Coon, 2007.	19 studies comparing three main EBT interventions covering PT (3), PE (14), and MC (2).	Studies only included in review if they demonstrated significant post-treatment effects and at least a small effect size. Largest effect was found for PT (all of which were CBT studies). Individual (not group) CBT for depression in caregivers is a very effective evidence-based treatment. Large effect effect size was also found for PE (especially if CBT-based), and moderate effect for the two MC interventions.	3 EBTs recommended for caregivers: PT, PE and MC. In the PE category there are 4 effective subtypes focused on depression, behaviour, anger and stress management. Largest effect and treatment outcome found for CBT interventions focused on CG depression.
Selwood et al., 2007.	62 evidence-based interventions with dementia caregivers examining efficacy of psychological treatments.	Few studies met quality criteria. Strongest evidence for individualised behavioural interventions. Group interventions less effective. Education by itself is not effective for CG depression, distress and burden. Coping strategy CG interventions strongest evidence for depression, inconsistent elsewhere. BM CG interventions are very varied. Evidence for group BM inconclusive. Individual BM is effective for depression in CG. Support group interventions non-effective.	Overall CG interventions have strongest impact on depression and less strong impact on burden. BM CG interventions are very varied. Evidence for group BM less strong than that for individual BM. The BM interventions often include a range of components, and may be better considered as CBT-oriented MC interventions. Interventions that focused on the individual circumstances of CGs (i.e. individual BM) and include the family, were most effective.

(Continued)

TABLE 11.3 *(Continued)*

Authors	Level of analysis	Results	Conclusions
Cooper et al., 2007.	24 studies looking at interventions for anxiety in caregivers.	Anxiety is a much neglected topic area for dementia CGs. Although 24 studies were identified only 1 study had anxiety reduction as a primary outcome and that was the only study to demonstrate clinical effects. All studies were methodologically poor. Interventions mixed therapeutic modality with service-level interventions.	'Our most striking finding was the lack of high level evidence, with no study demonstrating sufficient power to detect a difference in anxiety levels. The only RCT to report a significant reduction in anxiety was also the only study in which the intervention was specifically targeted at anxiety' (that study used a mix of CBT and relaxation strategies) (Cooper et al., 2007: 187).
Pinquart and Sorensen, 2011.	168 studies comparing spouse and non-spouse dementia caregivers, and included 19 studies looking at caregiving for physically frail older adults.	Large meta-analysis reveals significant differences between spouse and non-spouse CGs. Spouses were more likely to have higher depression scores. Low educational attainment, younger age, lower levels of informal support, being in employment and being in receipt of support were also associated with elevated depression scores.	'The present meta-analysis reveals considerable differences between spousal caregivers and adult children/children-in-law, the largest being on sociodemographic characteristics, such as age, marital status, employment status, and co-residence. In addition, spouses use less informal support, perceive their physical health to be worse, provide more care, and experience more depressive symptoms than do children and children-in-law' (Pinquart and Sorensen, 2011: 7).
Chien et al., 2011.	30 studies published between 1998 and 2009 were included in analyses looking at the efficacy of group-based support interventions for informal caregivers.	Multiple effect sizes were calculated from each study included in the review with an overall effect size averaged for each study. Studies included in the review focussed on different outcomes (well-being, burden, depression, social outcome). Multiple effect sizes were calculated for each outcome variable, although all reported significant effects for group-based caregiver interventions. Females tended to respond better to interventions. All effects were reduced at follow-up, although length of follow-up was variable.	'Support groups are significantly effective for caregivers of patients with dementia, while the effect size varies with different outcome variables, including psychological well-being, depression, burden and social outcomes. This finding proves that support groups are beneficial for caregivers of demented patients.' (Chien et al., 2011; P1097).

Authors	Level of analysis	Results	Conclusions
Vernooij-Dassen et al., 2011.	Cochrane Review looking at cognitive reframing (restructuring of negative appraisals) in caregivers of people with dementia. 11 RCT studies met criteria for inclusion. Caregivers included spouse and family carers. Included studies utilised stress-coping, stress behavioural and cognitive-behavioural treatment models.	2 out of 4 studies on anxiety show positive benefits of cognitive-reframing. Overall pooled results show positive impact on reducing anxiety. 4 out of 6 studies on depression show positive impact of cognitive reframing with an overall pooling of results suggesting this intervention is effective in reducing depression in caregivers. 3 out of 4 studies on caregiver distress reported positive effects of cognitive reframing in reducing distress, with overall pooled results favouring this intervention in reducing distress.	'This systematic review and meta-analysis of cognitive-reframing for family carers of persons with dementia showed beneficial effects over usual care for psychological morbidity (anxiety, depression) and (dis)stress. No effects were found for coping or self-efficacy, carer burden reaction to the relative's behaviour and institutionalization' (Vernooij-Dassen et al., 2011: 10).
Brodaty and Arasaratnam, 2012.	Reviewed the efficacy of non-pharmacological (psychosocial) interventions used with community-dwelling CGs managing psychological and behavioural symptoms of dementia. 23 papers published from 1985 to 2010 collected together 3,279 dyadic participants. 10/23 studies comment on follow-up of between 3–24 months after entry into individual trials.	The methodological quality of studies varied with 16/23 utilising a randomised controlled trial approach. There was a high level of variability in primary intervention approach with Brodaty and Arasaratnam (2012) categorising treatments as follows: skills training, education for CG, activity planning and environmental design, enhancing support for CGs, self-care techniques for CGs and miscellaneous. There was heterogeneity among studies in terms of participants and sample sizes across studies varied. The authors note that while successful interventions were home-based individualised (multicomponent) interventions tailored to the needs of the person with dementia and their CG, questions about optimal frequency, duration, intensity and location for treatments remain.	'This meta-analysis reveals that caregiver interventions can significantly reduce behavioral and psychological symptoms in the person with dementia as well as the caregiver's negative reactions to these symptoms.' (Brodaty and Arasaratnam, 2012: 948).

Notes: BM = Behavioural Management/Modification; CG = Caregivers (dementia); EBT = Evidence-based Treatment; MC = Multicomponent; PE = Psychoeducation; PT = Psychotherapy; PwD = Person with Dementia; RCT = Randomised Controlled Trial.

Health Administration and provides a very up-to-date systematic review of the evidence base of interventions aimed at non-professional carers (informal caregivers). In the UK, Elvish et al. (2012) have produced a report examining the evidence for psychosocial interventions with caregivers, and makes a series of sound recommendations for counsellors and psychotherapists contemplating working with caregivers.

Strong evidence for CBT for dementia can be found in dementia caregiver studies. A number of systematic reviews have demonstrated that CBT is an efficacious approach. Table 11.3 provides a snapshot of data, with regard to CBT-based caregiver interventions with evidence suggesting moderate effect size of CBT for dementia caregiver intervention outcome.

Overall the evidence for dementia caregiving suggests that interventions are more effective when they are active rather than passive. While psychoeducation improves subjective well-being, it is effective in reducing distress only if it is active. CBT works best when used on a more focal target such as reducing caregiver distress and burden. Consistent with the evidence for CBT for late life depression (see Chapter 3), individual interventions appear more effective than group interventions. Finally, as dementia is a deteriorating condition, interventions that are focused on one target may be less effective overall, and this is reflected in findings that only structured multi-component interventions are effective in reducing and delaying institutionalisation

Working with Dementia Caregivers Using CBT: Reasons for Caring

There are lots of reasons why carers do what they do. Some carers do this because of a sense of obligation, others may have a sense of reciprocity, or they might simply do it because they wouldn't want anyone else to care for their relative. When working with caregivers it may be a good idea to understand the reasons why their client decided to provide care.

Caregiving in dementia can have a negative impact on health, employment and, consequently, financial security (Alzheimer's Association, 2011). A report by the ILC in the UK noted that carers who provide more than 20 hours of care per week are more likely to either give up their job or reduce to part-time hours. It doesn't necessarily follow that providing care for someone with dementia is invariably perceived as burdensome or results in distress. Cohen et al. (2002) interviewed 289 carers and found that 73 per cent were able to identify at least one positive aspect of providing care, with 7 per cent able to find more than one positive experience of caring. Companionship and a sense of fulfilment/reward for providing care was most often mentioned (Cohen et al., 2002). Unsurprisingly, carers reporting more positive aspects of caregiving were at a lower risk of developing depression. Brodaty and Donkin (2009) suggest that positive and negative reasons for caring produce different emotional consequences for the carer. Caregivers who endorse more positive reasons for providing care unsurprisingly report experiencing less stress and feel more supported. Thus, therapists working with caregivers may wish to ask their clients: 'what are the reasons you care for your loved one?'

Guilt and Sense of Responsibility

Caregivers often have a strong sense of responsibility for providing care to their loved one. This can be a personally important motivation but it can also become an exhausting one, especially if a caregiver starts to neglect their own needs in order to provide care. Sometimes carers experience a whole set of conflicting emotions about the person they are caring for that makes them feel guilty. Perhaps they feel guilty when they want to have a break from being the strong one, or perhaps they feel ashamed of the thought that it would be better for their loved one to be dead, enters their head. When carers are stressed and tired they may be especially prone to having these thoughts and they feel very ashamed. It can be useful to have some way to capture this in therapy, and now therapists can utilise some new caregiver measures designed by psychotherapy researchers in Spain and validated for use with a UK sample (Roach et al., 2013). The Caregiver Guilt Questionnaire (Losada et al., 2010) and Dysfunctional Thoughts about Caregiving Questionnaire (Montorio et al., 2009) are ideally suited for use in CBT.

It is important to remind caregivers that they will experience many different emotions and thoughts, and that even ideas that they may feel disgusted by will enter their heads. It may be helpful for the therapist to acknowledge this fact and let the client know there is a word for these types of thoughts: *ego-dystonic*, meaning thoughts that are morally repugnant to us. We may try to suppress these thoughts, but that is ineffectual. However, you can remind your client of this simple truth: *thoughts are not facts, if you think something it is not morally the same as doing it.*

Case Example

Susan looks after her father Eric, who has recently been diagnosed with dementia. Her father also has cancer and has been told that this is untreatable. Susan's father, who has a mixed Alzheimer's and vascular dementia, appears to have poor insight into his condition but is also quite weepy when thinking about the future. It is uncertain how much information Eric has retained about his cancer diagnosis. Susan has said that her aim is to make her dad's experience with dementia as smooth as possible. When asked about her responsibility when caring for her dad she replies: 'I'm 100 per cent responsible for making sure his last months are comfortable.'

Reflection Point

Pause for a moment. Look at the above verbatim statement and think yourself into the situation.

Can you identify aspects of the situation Susan can control and aspects she cannot? For example, her own reaction to events may be under her control,

(Continued)

(Continued)

but how fast the deterioration in dementia will be and what form it will take is unknowable for anyone. The reaction of Susan's dad to events is also not under Susan's control.

What is the logical extension of her thoughts about caregiving?

You may notice that this statement has the hallmarks of a negative automatic thought. It is plausible, appears to be realistic and pro-social, coherent, persistent and perpetuating. It is also achievable, but only at great cost. It is likely to cause more distress and become self-defeating.

Evidently this is a very challenging task that Susan has set for herself, as she says she is convinced her dad doesn't like her because she is the only one that knows the true extent of his memory problems. Susan and Eric have found it difficult to agree on a number of solutions to problems. The therapist discussed with Susan the impact of believing she was 100 per cent responsible in this situation, especially as she may not have 100 per cent control of the situation or the future. When the responsibility pie was drawn at 100 per cent, Susan could quickly see this was unrealistic and added two pieces to the pie – her father and healthcare professionals – as others with responsibility for her father's experience with dementia. This was still an imbalance, as there are

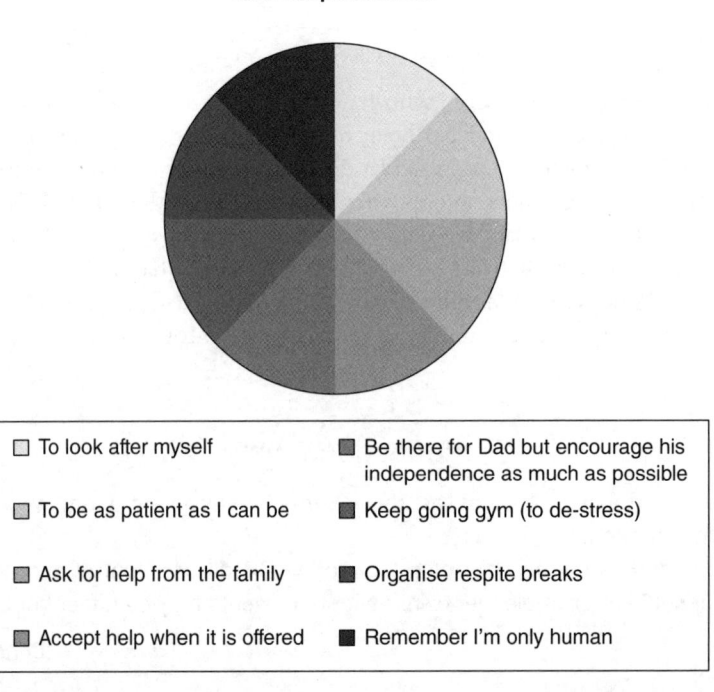

New Responsibilites

☐ To look after myself

☐ To be as patient as I can be

☐ Ask for help from the family

■ Accept help when it is offered

■ Be there for Dad but encourage his independence as much as possible

■ Keep going gym (to de-stress)

■ Organise respite breaks

■ Remember I'm only human

FIGURE 11.2 *New responsibilities pie chart*

many who can contribute to ensuring her father's last few months are comfortable and for ensuring that her father's current experience with dementia is as smooth as possible.

The aim here is not to absolve Susan of responsibility, but to allow her to focus her energy where she can be most helpful. The therapist asked about others who may have some responsibility. She was able to add her husband and her uncle. The therapist used the pie chart to discuss the idea of a backup team (see Figure 11.2). Susan was able to

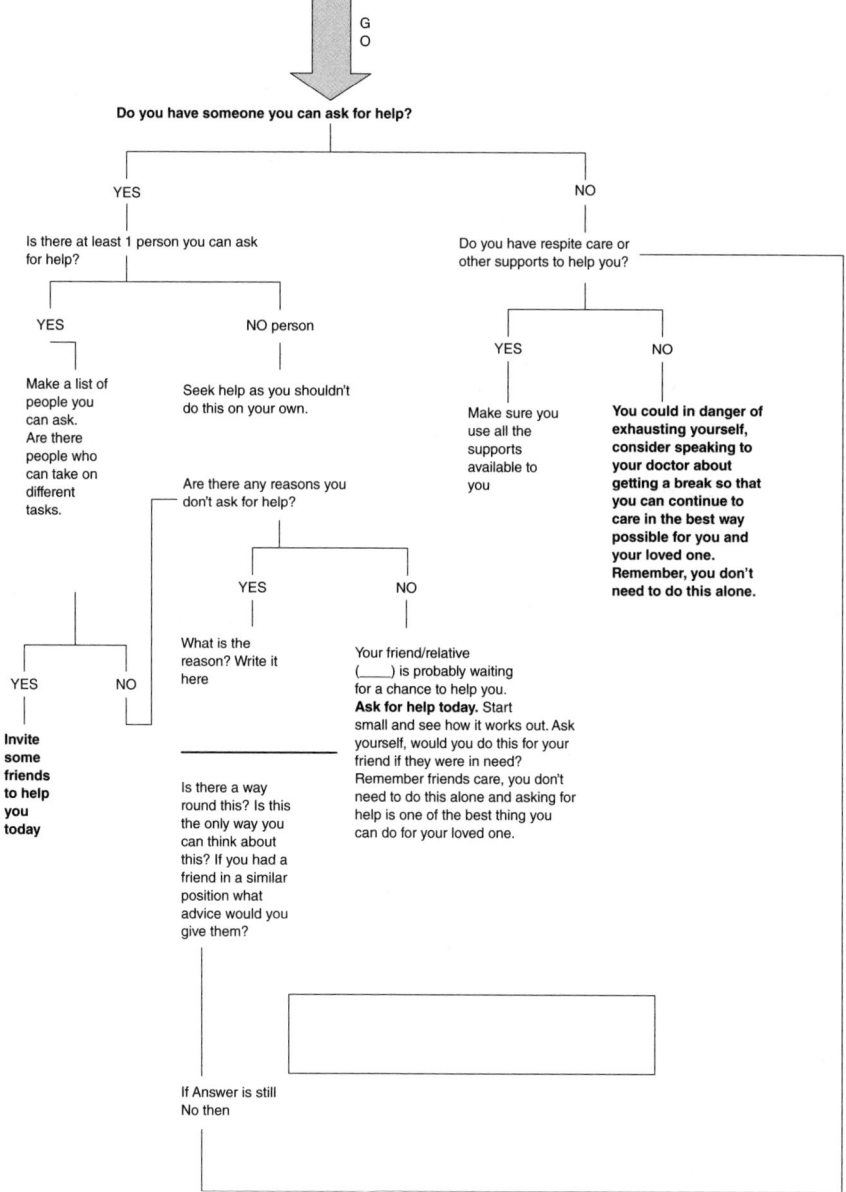

FIGURE 11.3   *Caregiving Help decision-tree*

A copy of this figure is available to download from https://study.sagepub.com/laidlaw

go from being 100 per cent responsible for providing care to developing a backup team that included her aunt, uncle, neighbour, husband and appropriate support services.

Asking for Help

Caregivers often find it difficult asking for others to help. There may be a number of reasons for this. Whatever reason the carer has for taking on caregiving tasks, it can be helpful in therapy if the client considers how they could seek assistance, and understands that to do so is neither a sign of weakness or failure, nor a lack of fulfilment of their commitment.

You might want to use the help decision-tree in Figure 11.3 to work out who your client could ask for help and what obstacles there are to doing so. It is important to destigmatise this, as you want to ensure that your client has an acceptable rationale about receiving help. You may wish to remind your client that *in order to care for their loved ones they need to care for themselves.* You might want to use an athlete analogy. An athlete can achieve only so much on their own – without a coach and a backup team they are likely to fail. In the meantime you (the therapist) can act as the coach, but they still will need a backup team. It is not weak or wrong to ask for help – it is a normal human response to a potentially difficult situation.

Summary and Conclusions

As people live longer, there will be relatively large numbers of older people who experience dementia because of the increase in longevity rather than an epidemic in dementia. For the majority of older people, however, growing older is a surprisingly positive experience, and the evidence suggests that older people report high levels of life satisfaction, are better at emotional regulation strategies and have better emotional stability. The structured nature of CBT sessions may make it particularly helpful to those whose memory abilities are compromised, and may be especially relevant in treating depression in dementia, with a focus on practical and pragmatic problem solving.

Giving people a chance to reflect on the meaning of a life-changing and life-threatening diagnosis such as dementia, and to work collaboratively and proactively to promote the highest possible levels of functional independence, seems to be a very important opportunity for society to provide for its most vulnerable members.

Learning Log: Reflection and Review
What have you gained from reading this chapter?

- Think about the different types of dementia, and in particular think about how this influences how you work with your clients and how their needs may differ. If you were to consider adaptations they may include ways to enhance recall between sessions.

- Think about the structured nature of CBT and whether this may enhance the accessibility of psychological therapy.
- As a dementia diagnosis has implications and ramifications for many people and not just the person receiving the diagnosis, consider what the unique and the complimentary needs of the person with dementia and their primary caregiver will be. Is it possible to reconcile this in a single treatment intervention?
- Look at the empirical evidence, think about the gaps in the knowledge and consider what implications this may have on your practice.
- Reflect on the standard techniques in CBT for use with caregivers, and reflect on how these are translated into your own routine practice.

Further Reading

The following sources provide more in-depth coverage of topics raised in this chapter.

James, I. A. (2010). *Cognitive behavioural therapy with older people: interventions for those with and without dementia*. London: Jessica Kingsley.

Elvish, R., Lever, S-J., Johnstone, J., Cawley, R., & Keady, J. (2012). *Psychological interventions for carers of people with dementia: a systematic review of quantitative and qualitative evidence*. London: BACP UK.

References

Aarsland, D., Cumming, J. L., & Larsen, J. P. (2001). Neuropsychiatric differences between Parkinson's disease with dementia and Alzheimer's disease. *International Journal of Geriatric Psychiatry, 16,* 184–191.

Achenbaum, W. A. (2013). Robert N. Butler (January 21, 1927–July 4, 2010): visionary leader. *The Gerontologist, 53,* 1–7.

Alexopoulous, G. S. (2005). Depression in the elderly. *Lancet, 365,* 1961–1970.

Alexopoulos, G. S., Abrams, R. C., Young, R. C., & Shamoian, C. A. (1988). Cornell Scale for Depression in Dementia. *Biological Psychiatry, 23*(3), 271–284.

ADI, Alzheimer's Disease International (2012). *World Alzheimer report 2012: overcoming the stigma of dementia.* London: ADI. Available at: www.alz.co.uk/research/WorldAlzheimerReport2012.pdf

Alzheimer's Association (2011). Alzheimer's Association report 2011: Alzheimer's disease facts and figures. *Alzheimer's and Dementia, 7,* 208–244.

Alzheimer's Society (2011). *Optimising treatment and care for people with behavioural and psychological symptoms of dementia: a best practice guide for health and social care professionals.* London: Alzheimer's Society.

APA, American Psychiatric Association (2000). *Diagnostic and Statistical Manual of Mental Disorders,* Fourth Edition, Text Revision (DSM-IV-TR). Washington, DC: American Psychiatric Association.

APA, American Psychiatric Association (2013). Highlight of changes from DSM-IV-TR to DSM-5. Available at: www.dsm5.org/Documents/changes%20from%20dsm-iv-tr%20to%20%20dsm-5.pdf

Aspinall, A. (2013). *Is cognitive behavioural therapy as efficacious in treating generalised anxiety disorder in older people compared to adults of working age?* Unpublished MSc by research dissertation, University of Edinburgh.

Ayers, C. R., Sorrell, J. T., Thorp, S. R., & Wetherell, J. L. (2007). Evidence-based psychological treatments for late life anxiety. *Psychology & Aging, 22,* 8–17.

Baltes, P. B. & Kunzmann, U. (2004). The two faces of wisdom: wisdom as a general theory of knowledge and judgement about excellence in mind and virtue vs. wisdom as everyday realization in people and products. *Human Development, 47,* 290–299.

Baltes, P. B. & Smith, J. (2003). New frontiers in the future of aging: from successful aging of the young-old to the dilemmas of the fourth age. *Gerontology, 49,* 123–135.

Baltes, P. B. & Smith, J. (2008). The fascination of wisdom: its nature, ontogeny, and function, *Perspectives on Psychological Science, 3,* 56–64.

Baltes, P. B. & Staudinger, U. M. (2000). Wisdom: a metaheuristic (pragmatic) to orchestrate mind and virtue toward excellence. *American Psychologist, 55*, 122–136.

Baraniak, A. & Sheffield, D. (2011). The efficacy of psychologically based interventions to improve anxiety, depression and quality of life in COPD: a systematic review and meta-analysis, *Patient Education and Counseling, 83*, 29–36.

Barkham, M., Culverwell, A., Spindler, K., & Twigg, E. (2005). The CORE-OM in an older adult population: psychometric status, acceptability, and feasibility. *Aging & Mental Health, 9*, 235–245.

Barrowclough, C., King, P., Colville, J., Russell, E., Burns, A., & Tarrier, N. (2001) A randomized trial of the effectiveness of cognitive-behavioral therapy and supportive counselling for anxiety symptoms in older adults. *Journal of Consulting and Clinical Psychology, 69*, 756–762.

Bauer, J. & McAdams, D. (2004). Personal growth in adults' stories of life transitions. *Journal of Personality, 72*, 573–602.

Beck, A. T., Rush, A. J., Shaw, B. F., & Emery, G. (1979). *Cognitive therapy of depression.* New York: Guilford Press.

Beck A. T. (1976). *Cognitive therapy and the emotional disorders.* New York: Meridien.

Beck, A. T. (1983). Cognitive therapy of depression: New perspectives. In P. J. Clayton & J. E. Barrett (Eds.) *Treatment of depression: Old controversies and new approaches.* New York: Raven Press.

Beck, A. T. (2008). The evolution of the cognitive model of depression and its neurobiological correlates. *The American Journal of Psychiatry, 165*, 969–977.

Beck, A. T., Epstein, N., Brown, G. K., & Steer, R. A. (1988). An inventory for measuring clinical anxiety: psychometric properties. *Journal of Consulting and Clinical Psychology, 56*, 893–897.

Beck, A. T., Steer, R. A., & Brown, G. K. (1996). *The Beck Depression Inventory-II.* San Antonio, TX: Psychological Corporation.

Beck, J. S. (2011). *Cognitive behavior therapy: basics and beyond* (2nd ed.). New York: Guilford Press.

Beck, R. & Perkins, T. S. (2001). Cognitive content-specificity for anxiety and depression: a meta analysis. *Cognitive Therapy and Research, 25*, 651–663.

Beekman, A. T., Copeland, J. R. M., & Prince, M. J. (1999). Review of community prevalence of depression in later life. *British Journal of Psychiatry, 174*, 307–311.

Bishop, W. & Fish, J. M. (1999). Questions as interventions: Perceptions of Socratic, solution focused and diagnostic questioning styles. *Journal of Rational-Emotive and Cognitive-Behavior Therapy, 17*, 115–140.

Bjelland, I., Dahl, A. A., Haug, T. T., & Neckelmann, D. (2002). The validity of the Hospital and Anxiety Depression Scale: an updated literature review. *Journal of Psychosomatic Research, 52*, 69–77.

Blackburn, I. M., James, I. A., Milne, D. L., Baker, C., Standart, S., Garland, A., & Reichelt, F. K. (2001). The revised cognitive therapy scale (CTS-R): psychometric properties. *Behavioural and Cognitive Psychotherapy, 29*, 431–446.

Blazer, D. (2010). Protection from late life depression. *International Psychogeriatrics, 22*, 171–173.

Blazer, D. G. & Hybels, C. F. (2005). Origins of depression in later life. *Psychological Medicine, 35*, 1–12.

Blenkiron, P. (1999). Who is suitable for cognitive behavioural therapy? *Journal of the Royal Society of Medicine, 92*, 222–229.

Bluck, S. & Glück, J. (2004). Making things better and learning a lesson: experiencing wisdom across the lifespan. *Journal of Personality, 72*, 543–572.

Boddice, G., Pachana, N. A., & Byrne, G. J. (2008). The clinical utility of the Geriatric Anxiety Inventory in older adults with cognitive impairment. *Nursing Older People, 20*, 36–39.

Bodner, E. (2009). On the origins of ageism among older and younger adults. *International Psychogeriatrics, 21*, 1003–1014.

Bohner, G. & Dickel, N. (2011). Attitudes and attitude change. *Annual Review of Psychology, 62*, 391–417.

Bonder, B. R. (1994). Psychotherapy for individuals with Alzheimer disease. *Alzheimer Disease and Associated Disorders, 8*, (Suppl. 3), 75–81.

Bondi, M. W., Salmon, D. P., & Kaszniak, A. W. (2009). The neuropsychology of dementia. In I. Grant & K. M. Adams (Eds.), *Neuropsychological assessment of neuropsychiatric and neuromedical disorders* (pp. 159–198). New York: Oxford University Press.

Brodaty, H. (2003). Meta-analysis of psychosocial interventions for caregivers of people with dementia. *Journal of the American Geriatric Society, 51*, 657–664.

Brodaty, H. & Arasaratnam, C. (2012). Meta-analysis of nonpharmacological symptoms of dementia. *American Journal of Psychiatry, 169*, 946–953.

Brodaty, H. & Donkin, M. (2009). Family caregivers of people with dementia. *Dialogues in Clinical NeuroSciences, 11*, 217–228.

Broomfield, N., Laidlaw, K., Hickabottom, E., Murray, M., Pendrey, R., Whittick, J., & Gillespie, D. (2011). Post-stroke depression: The case for augmented Cognitive Behaviour Therapy. *Clinical Psychology & Psychotherapy: An International Journal of Theory & Practice, 18* (3), 202–218.

Bryant, C., Bei, B., Gilson, K., Komiti, A., Jackson, H., & Judd, F. (2012). The relationship between attitudes to aging and physical and mental health in older adults. *International Psychogeriatrics, 24*, 1674–1683.

Bryant, C., Jackson, H., & Ames, D. (2008). The prevalence of anxiety in older adults: methodological issues and a review of the literature. *Journal of Affective Disorders, 109*, 233–250.

Burroughs, H., Lovell, K., Morley, M., Baldwin, R., Burns, A., & Chew-Graham, C. (2006). 'Justifiable depression': How primary care professionals and patients view late life depression? A qualitative study. *Family Practice, 23*, 369–377.

Byrne, G. J. & Pachana, N. A. (2010). Development and validation of a short form of the Geriatric Anxiety Inventory: The GAI-SF. *International Psychogeriatrics, 22*, 5.

Caputo, M., Monstero, R., Mariani, E., Santucci, A., Mangialasche, F., Camardi, R., Senin, U., & Mecocci, P. (2008). Neuropsychiatric symptoms in 921 elderly subjects with dementia: a comparison between vascular and neurodegenerative types. *Acta Psychiatrica Scandinavica, 117*, 455–464.

Carstensen, L. L. & Lockenhoff, C. A. (2003). Aging, emotion, and evolution: The bigger picture. *Annals of the New York Academy of Sciences, 1000*, 152–179.

Carstensen, L. L., Turan, B., Scheibe, S., Ram, N., Erser-Hershfeld, H., Samanez-Larkin, G., Brooks, K. P., & Nesselroade, J. R. (2011). Emotional experience improves with age: evidence based on over 10 years of experience sampling. *Psychology and Aging, 26*, 21–33.

Carstensen, L. L., Fung, H. H., & Charles, S. T. (2003). Socioemotional selectivity theory and the regulation of emotion in the second half of life. *Motivation and Emotion, 27*, 103–123.

Carstensen, L. L., Isaacowitz, D., & Charles, S. T. (1999). Taking time seriously: a theory of socioemotional selectivity. *American Psychologist, 54*, 165–181.

Chachamovich, E., Fleck, M., Laidlaw, K., & Power, M. (2008). Impact of major depression and subsyndromal symptoms on quality of life and attitudes toward aging in an international sample of older adults. *Gerontologist, 48*, 593–602.

Charidimou, A., Seamons, J., Selai, C., & Schrag, A. (2011). The role of cognitive-behavioural therapy for patients with depression in Parkinson's disease. *Parkinson's disease*, article ID 737523, doi:10.4061/2011/737523.

Charlesworth, G. & Greenfield, S. (2004). Overcoming barriers to collaborative conceptualization in cognitive therapy with older adults. *Behavioural and Cognitive Psychotherapy, 32*, 411–422.

Chien, L., Chu, H., Guo, J., Liao, Y., Chang, L., Chen, C., & Chou, K. (2011). Caregiver support groups in patients with dementia: a meta-analysis. *International Journal of Geriatric Psychiatry, 26*(10), 1089–1098.

Cinamon, J. S., Finch, L., Miller, S., Higgins, J., & Mayo, N. (2010). Preliminary evidence for the development of a stroke specific geriatric depression scale. *International Journal of Geriatric Psychiatry, 26*, 188–198.

Clark, D. A., Beck, A. T., & Alford, B. A. (1999). *Scientific foundations of cognitive theory and therapy of depression*. New York: Guilford Press.

Cohen, J. (1992). A power primer. *Psychological Bulletin, 112*, 155–159.

Cohen, C. A., Colantonio, A., & Vernich, L. (2002). Positive aspects of caregiving: rounding out the caregiver experience. *International Journal of Geriatric Psychiatry, 17*, 184–188.

Cooke, D. D., McNally, L., Mulligan, K. T., Harrison, M. J. G., & Newman, S. P. (2001). Psychosocial interventions for caregivers of people with dementia: A systematic review. *Aging & Mental Health, 5*, 120–135.

Coon, D. W. & Gallagher-Thompson, D. (2002) Encouraging homework completion among older adults in therapy. *JCLP/In session: Psychotherapy in Practice, 58*, 549–563.

Cooper, C., Balamurali, T., & Livingston, G. (2007). A systematic review of the prevalence and associates of anxiety in caregivers of people with dementia. *International Psychogeriatrics, 19*, 175–195.

Crittendon, J. & Hopko, D. R. (2006). Assessing worry in older and younger adults: psychometric properties of an abbreviated Penn State Worry Questionnaire (PDWQ-A). *Journal of Anxiety Disorders, 20*, 1036–1054.

Cuijpers, P., van Straten, A., Smit, F., & Andersson, G. (2009). Is psychotherapy for depression equally effective in younger and in older adults? A meta-regression analysis. *International Psychogeriatrics, 21*, 16–24.

D'Ath, P., Katona, P., Mullan, E., Evans, S., & Katona, C. (1994). Screening, detection and management of depression in primary care attenders I: the acceptability and performance of the 15 item Geriatric Depression Scale (GDS15) and the development of shorter versions. *Family Practice, 11,* 260–266.

Debruyne, H., Van Buggenhout, M., et al. (2009). Is the geriatric depression scale a reliable screening tool for depressive symptoms in elderly patients with cognitive impairment? *International Journal of Geriatric Psychiatry, 24,* 556–562.

DEMOS (2012). *Ageing across Europe: a report prepared by DEMOS for WRVS May 2012.* Cardiff: WRVS.

Dennis, R. E., Boddington, S. J. A., & Funnell, N. J. (2007). Self-report measures of anxiety: are they suitable for older adults? *Aging & Mental Health, 11,* 668–677.

Dennis, M., Kadri, A., & Coffey, J. (2012). Depression in older people in the general hospital: a systematic review of screening instruments. *Age & Ageing, 41,* 148–154.

Diefenbach, G. J. & Goethe, J. (2006). Clinical interventions for late-life anxious depression. *Clinical Interventions in Aging, 1,* 41–50.

Diehl, M. K. & Werner-Wahl, H. (2010). Awareness of age-related change: examination of a (mostly) unexplored concept. *Journals of Gerontology Series B: Psychological Sciences and Social Sciences, 65,* 340–350.

Dobkin, R. D., Menza, M., Allen, L. A., Gara, M. A., Margery, M. H., Tiu, J., Bienfait, K. L., & Friedman, J. (2011). Cognitive-behavioral therapy for depression in Parkinson's disease: A randomized controlled trial. *The American Journal of Psychiatry, 168,* 1066–1074.

Dryden, W. (2009). The importance of choice in therapy: from the perspective of a, hopefully flexible, CBT practitioner. *European Journal of Psychotherapy and Counselling, 11,* 311–322.

Dryden, W. & Branch, R. (Eds.). (2012). *The CBT handbook.* London: SAGE.

Edelstein, B. A., Woodhead, E. L., Segal, D. L., Heisel, M. J., Bower, E. H., Lowery, A. J., & Stoner, S. A. (2008). Older adult psychological assessment: current instrument status and related circumstances. *Clinical Gerontologist, 31,* 1–35.

Ell, K., Unutzer, J., Aranda, M., Snachez, K., & Lee, P-J. (2005). Routine PHQ-9 depression screening in home health care: depression prevalence, clinical and treatment characteristics and screening implementation. *Home Health Care Services Quarterly, 24,* 1–19.

Elvish, R., Lever, S-J., Johnstone, J., Cawley, R., & Keady, J. (2012). *Psychological interventions for carers of people with dementia: a systematic review of quantitative and qualitative evidence.* London: BACP UK.

Enache, D., Winblad, B., & Aarsland, D. (2011). Depression in dementia: epidemiology, mechanisms, and treatment. *Current Opinion in Psychiatry, 24,* 461–472.

Ertan, F.S., Ertan, T., Kiziltan, G. & Uygucgil, H. (2005) Reliability and validity of the Geriatric Depression Scale in depression in Parkinson's disease. *J. Neurol. Neurosurg. Psychiatry, 76,* 1445-1447.

Faraone, S.V. (2008). Interpreting estimates of treatment effects: implications for managed care. *Pharmacy & Therapeutics, 33,* 700–711.

Fletcher, E. H., Woodford, H. J., & George, J. (2007). Assessment of suspected dementia in older people. *Reviews in Clinical Gerontology, 17,* 63–73.

Fries, J. F. (2003). Measuring and monitoring success in compressing morbidity. *Annals Internal Medicine, 139,* 455–459.

Freund, A. (2008). Successful aging as management of resources: the role of selection, optimization, and compensation. *Research in Human Development, 5,* 94–106.

Freund, A. & Baltes, P. (1998). Selection, optimization, and compensation as strategies of life-management: correlations with subjective indicators of successful aging. *Psychology & Aging, 13,* 531–543.

Frijters, P. & Beatton, T. (2012). The mystery of the U-shaped relationship between happiness and age. *Journal of Economic Behavior & Organization, 82,* 525–542.

Fry, P. S. (1986). *Depression, stress and adaptations in the elderly: Psychological assessment and intervention.* Rockville, MD: Aspen.

Gallagher-Thompson, D. & Coon, D. W. (2007). Evidence-based psychological treatments for distress in family caregivers of older adults. *Psychology and Aging, 22*(1), 37–51.

Garratt, G., Ingram, R. E., Rand, K. L., & Sawalani, G. (2007). Cognitive processes in cognitive therapy: evaluation of the mechanisms of change in the treatment of depression. *Clinical Psychology: Science and Practice, 14,* 224–239.

Germer, C. K. & Siegel, R. D. (Eds.). (2012). *Wisdom and compassion in psychotherapy: deepening mindfulness in clinical practice.* New York: Guilford Press Inc.

Gloster, A. T., Rhoades, H. M., Novy, D., Klotsche, J., Senior, A., Kunik, M., Wilson, N., & Stanley, M. A. (2008). Psychometric properties of the Depression Anxiety and Stress Scale-21 in older primary care patients. *Journal of Affective Disorders, 110,* 248–259.

Goncalves, D. & Byrne, G. (2012). Interventions for generalized anxiety disorders in older adults: systematic review and meta-analysis. *Journal of Anxiety Disorders, 26,* 1–11.

Gorenstein, E. E. & Papp, L. A. (2007). Cognitive behavior therapy for anxiety in the elderly. *Current Psychiatry Reports, 9,* 20–25.

Gotlib, I. H. & Joormann, J. (2010) Cognition and depression: Current status and future directions. *Annual Review of Clinical Psychology, 6,* 285–312.

Gould, R. L., Coulson, M. C., & Howard, R. J. (2012a). Cognitive behavioral therapy for depression in older people: a meta-analysis and meta-regression of randomized controlled trials. *Journal of the American Geriatric Society, 60,* 1817–1830.

Gould, R. L., Coulson, M. C., & Howard, R. J. (2012b). Cognitive behavioral therapy for anxiety disorders in older people: a meta-analysis and meta-regression of randomized controlled trials. *Journal of the American Geriatric Society, 60,* 218–229.

Gotlib, I. H., Krasnoperova, E., Neubauer Yue, D., & Joorman, J. (2004). Attentional bias for negative interpersonal stimuli in clinical depression. *Journal of Abnormal Psychology, 113,* 127–135.

Gotlib, I. H., & Joormann, J. (2010). Cognition and depression: current status and future directions. *Annual Review of Clinical Psychology, 6,* 285–312.

Goy, E., Freeman, M., & Kansagara, D. (2010). A Systematic Evidence Review of Interventions for Non-professional Caregivers of Individuals with Dementia. VA-ESP Project #05-225.

Grant, R. W. & Casey, D. A. (1995). Adapting cognitive behavioral therapy for the frail elderly. *International Psychogeriatrics, 7,* 561-571

Gum, A., Arean, P., Hunkeler, E., Tang, L., Katon, W., Hitchcock, P., Steffens, D., Dickens, J., & Unutzer, J. (2006). Depression treatment preferences in older primary care patients. *The Gerontologist, 46,* 14–22.

Gupta, S. K. (2011). Intention to treat concept: A review. *Perspectives in Clinical Research, 2,* 109–112.

Hackett, M. L., Yapa, C., Parag, V., & Anderson, C. S. (2005). Frequency of depression after stroke: A systematic review of observational studies. *Stroke, 36,* 1330–1340.

Haringsma, R., Engels, G. I., Beekman, A. T. F., & Spinhaven, P. (2004). The criterion validity of the Center for Epidemiological Studies Depression Scale (CES-D) in a sample of self-referred elders with depressive symptomatology. *International Journal of Geriatric Psychiatry*, *19*, 558–563.

Hendriks, G., Oude, R., Voshaar, G., et al. (2008). Cognitive-behavioural therapy for late-life anxiety disorder: A systematic review and meta-analysis. *Acta Psychiatrica Scandinavica*, *117*, 403–411.

Higgins, E. T. (1987). Self-discrepancy: a theory relating self and affect. *Psychological Review*, *94*, 319–340.

Hinrichsen, G. (2010) Sexual orientation issues in the context of interpersonal therapy for late life depression. In N. A. Pachana, K. Laidlaw & B. G. Knight (Eds.) *Casebook of clinical geropsychology: International perspectives on practice*. Oxford: OUP. pp. 1–14.

Hoffman, S. G. & Smits, J. A. J. (2008). Cognitive-behavioral therapy for adult anxiety disorders: A meta-analysis of randomized placebo-controlled trials. *Journal of Clinical Psychiatry*, *69*, 621–632.

Hollon, S. D. & Ponniah, K., (2010). A review of empirically supported psychological therapies for mood disorders in adults. *Depression and Anxiety*, *27*, 891–932.

House of Lords (2013). *Ready for Ageing? Report*. Select Committee on Public Service and Demographic Change. Report of Session 2012–13. London: The Stationery Office.

Hunot, V., Churchill, R., Teixeira, V., & Silva de Lima, M. (2007). Psychological therapies for generalized anxiety disorder. *Cochrane Database of Systematic Reviews*, *1*, CD001848. DOI: 10.1002/14651858.CD001848.pub4.

Hunot, V., Churchill, R., Teixeira, V., & Silva de Lima, M. (2010). Psychological therapies for generalized anxiety disorder. Cochrane Database of Systematic Reviews, 1, CD001848. DOI: 10.1002/14651858.CD001848.pub4.

Hyer, L., Kramer, D., & Sohnle, S. (2004). CBT with older people: alterations and the value of the therapeutic alliance. *Psychotherapy: Theory, Research, Practice, Training*, *41*, 276–291.

Hynninen, M. J., Bjerke, N., Pallesen, S., Bakke, P. S., & Hilde Nordhus, I. (2010). A randomized controlled trial of cognitive behavioural therapy for anxiety and depression in COPD. *Respiratory Medicine*, *104*, 986–994.

IAPT (2008). *Long-term conditions positive practice guide*. London: DOH.

Izal, M., Montario, I., Nuevo, R., Pereze-Rojo, G., & Cabrera, I. (2010). Optimising the diagnostic performance of the Geriatric Depression Scale. *Psychiatry Research*, *178*, 142–146.

Jakobsons, L. J., Brown, J. S., Gordon, K. H., & Joiner, T. E. (2007). When are clients ready to terminate? *Cognitive and Behavioral Practice*, *24*(2), 218–230.

Johnson, H. (2013). We will be different! Ageism and the temporal construction of old age. *The Getontologist*, *53*, 198–204.

Joorman, J., Teachman, B. A., & Gotlib, I. H. (2009). Sadder and less accurate? False memory for negative material in depression. *Journal of Abnormal Psychology*, *118*, 412–417.

Jorm, A. F. (2000). Does old age reduce the risk of anxiety and depression? A review of epidemiological studies across the life span. *Psychological Medicine*, *30*, 11–12.

Karel, M. J., Gatz, M., & Smyer, M. A. (2012). Aging and mental health in the decade ahead: what psychologists need to know. *American Psychologist, 67*, 184–198.

Kazantzis, N., Deane, F. R., Ronan, K. R, & L'Abate, L. (2005). *Using homework assignments in cognitive behavior therapy*. New York: Routledge.

Kinderman, P. & Tai, S. (2007). Clinical implications of a psychological model of mental disorder. *Behavioural and Cognitive Psychotherapy, 35*, 1–14.

Kingdon, D., Hanse, L., Finn, M., & Turkington, D. (2007). When standard cognitive-behavioural therapy is not enough. *Psychiatric Bulletin, 31*, 121–123.

Kinsella, K. & Wan, H. (2009). *US Census Bureau, series P95/09–1, an ageing world: 2008*. Washington, DC: US Government Printing Office. Available at: www.census.gov/prod/2009pubs/p95–09–1.pdf

Kiosses, D., Teri, L., Velligan, D. L., & Alexopolous, G. (2011). A home-delivered intervention for depressed, cognitively impaired disabled elders. *International Journal of Geriatric Psychiatry, 26*, 256–262.

Kirschenbaum, H. & Henderson, V. L. (Eds.). (1990). *The Carl Rogers reader: selections from the lifetime work of America's preeminent psychologist, author of* On Becoming a Person *and* A Way of Being. London: Constable.

Kitwood, T. (1997). *Dementia reconsidered: The person comes first*. London: Open University Press (OUP).

Knight, B. G. (2004). *Psychotherapy with older adults* (3rd Edn). Thousand Oaks, CA: Sage Publications.

Knight, B. G. (2006). Unique aspects of psychotherapy with older adults. In S. Quall & B. G. Knight (Eds.), *Psychotherapy with older adults*. New York: John Wiley & Sons.

Knight, B. G., Karel, M. G., Hinrichsen, G. A., Qualls, S. H., & Duffy, M. (2009). Pike's Peak model for training in professional geropsychology. *American Psychologist, 64*, 205–214.

Knight, B. G. & Laidlaw, K. (2009). Translational theory: a wisdom-based model for psychological interventions to enhance well-being in later life. In V. Bengston, M. Silverstein, N. M. Putney, & D. Gans (Eds.), *Handbook of theories of aging* (2nd ed.). New York: Springer.

Koder, D. A. (1998). Treatment of anxiety in the cognitively impaired elderly: Can cognitive-behavior therapy help? *International Psychogeriatrics, 10*, 173–182.

Kraus, C. A., Seignourel, P., Balasubramanyam, V., Snow, L., Wilson, N. L., Kunik, M., Schulz, P., & Stanley, M. A. (2008). Cognitive-behavioral treatment for anxiety in patients with dementia: Two case studies. *Journal of Psychiatric Practice, 14*, 186–192.

Krishna, M., Jauhari, A., Lepping, P., Turner, J., Crossley, D., & Krishnamoorthy, A. (2011). Is group psychotherapy effective in older adults with depression? *International Journal of Geriatric Psychiatry, 26*, 331–340.

Krishnan, K. R. K., Delong, M., Kraemer, H., Carney, R., Spiegel, D., Gordon, C., et al. (2002). Comorbidity of depression with other medical diseases in the elderly. *Biological Psychiatry, 52*, 559–588.

Kroenke, K. & Spitzer, R. L. (2002). The PHQ-9: a new depression diagnostic and severity measure. *Psychiatric Annals, 32*, 1–7.

Kunik, M. E., Braun, U., Stanley, M. A., Wristers, K., Molinari, V., Stoebner, D., & Orengo, C. A. (2001). One session cognitive behavioural therapy for elderly patients with chronic obstructive pulmonary disease. *Psychological Medicine, 31*, 717–723.

Kunik, M. E., Veazey, C., Cully, J., Souchek, J., Graham, D. P., Hopko, D., Carter, R., Sharafkhaneh, A., Goepfert, E. J., Wray, N., & Stanley, M. A. (2008). COPD education and cognitive behavioural therapy group treatment for clinically significant symptoms of depression and anxiety in COPD: a randomized controlled trial. *Psychological Medicine, 38*, 385–396.

Kuruvilla, T., Fenwick, C. D., Haque, M. S., & Vassilas, C. A. (2006). Elderly depressed patients: what are their views on treatment options? *Aging & Mental Health, 10*, 204–206.

Kuyken, W. (2006) Digging deep into depression: the phenomenon of overgeneralised autobiographical memory in depression. *The Psychologist, 19*, 278–281.

Kuyken, W., Padesky, C. A., & Dudley, R. (2009). *Collaborative case conceptualization: working effectively with clients in cognitive behavioral therapy*. New York: Guilford Press.

Laidlaw, K. (2001) Cognitive therapy for late life depression: Does research evidence suggest adaptations are necessary for cognitive therapy with older adults? *Clinical Psychology & Psychotherapy: An International Journal of Theory & Practice, 8*, 1–14.

Laidlaw, K. (2008a). Cognitive behaviour therapy, in R. T. Woods & L. Clare (Eds.), *Handbook of the clinical psychology of ageing* (2nd Edn). Chichester: John Wiley & Sons Ltd.

Laidlaw, K. (2008b). Using CBT with older people with post-stroke depression. In D. Gallagher-Thompson, A. Steffen, & L. W. Thompson (Eds.), *Handbook of behavioral and cognitive therapies with older adults*. New York: John Wiley & Sons.

Laidlaw, K. (2008c). Cognitive behaviour therapy for depression in Parkinson's disease. In K. Laidlaw & B.G. Knight (Eds.), *Handbook of the assessment and treatment of emotional disorders in later life*. Oxford: Oxford University Press.

Laidlaw, K. (2010a). Are attitudes to ageing and wisdom enhancement legitimate targets for CBT for late life depression? *Nordic Psychology, 62*(2), 27–42.

Laidlaw, K. (2010b). Enhancing cognitive behaviour therapy with older people using gerontological theories as vehicles for change. In N. A. Pachana, K. Laidlaw, & B. G. Knight (Eds.), *Casebook of clinical geropsychology: international perspectives on practice*. Oxford: Oxford University Press.

Laidlaw, K. (2013a). Self-acceptance and aging: using self-acceptance as a mediator of change in CBT with depressed and anxious older people. In M. E. Bernard (Ed.), *The strength of self-acceptance*. Melbourne: Springer.

Laidlaw, K. (2013b). ViewPoint: a deficit in psychotherapeutic care for older people with depression and anxiety. *Gerontology: International Journal of Experimental, Clinical, Behavioural, Regenerative and Technological Gerontology*, DOI: 10.1159/000351439.

Laidlaw, K. (2013c). CBT for late life anxiety: not yet fulfilling its potential with older people? *DCP Clinical Psychology Forum (Newsletter), 250*, 18–24.

Laidlaw, K. & McAlpine, S. (2008). Cognitive-behaviour therapy: how is it different with older people? *Journal of Rational Emotive Cognitive Behaviour Therapy, 26*(4), 250–262.

Laidlaw, K. & Pachana, N. A. (2009). Aging, mental health, and demographic change: challenges for psychotherapists. *Professional Psychology: Research and Practice, 40*, 601–608.

Laidlaw, K. & Pachana, N. A. (2011). CE Corner: Aging with grace. *Monitor on Psychology*, Nov., 66–71.

Laidlaw, K. & Thompson, L. W. (2008). Cognitive Behaviour Therapy with Older People. In K. Laidlaw & B. G. Knight (Eds.), *Handbook of the assessment and treatment of emotional disorders in later life*. Oxford: Oxford University Press.

Laidlaw, K., Thompson, L. W., Siskin-Dick, L., & Gallagher-Thompson, D. (2003). *Cognitive behavioural therapy with older people*. Chichester: John Wiley & Sons.

Laidlaw, K., Thompson, L., & Gallagher-Thompson, D. (2004). Comprehensive conceptualisation of cognitive behaviour therapy for late life depression. *Behavioural & Cognitive Psychotherapy*, *32*, 1–11.

Laidlaw, K., Power, M. J., & Schmidt, S. (2007). The Attitudes to Ageing Questionnaire (AAQ): development and psychometric properties. *International Journal of Geriatric Psychiatry*, *22*, 367–379.

Laidlaw, K., Davidson, K. M., Toner, H. L., Jackson, G., Clark, S., Law, J., Howley, M., Bowie, G., & Connery, H. (2008). A randomised controlled trial of cognitive behaviour therapy versus treatment as usual in the treatment of mild to moderate late life depression. *International Journal of Geriatric Psychiatry*, *23*(8), 843–850.

Lee, D. R., Taylor, J-P., & Thomas, A. J. (2012). Assessment of cognitive fluctuation in dementia: a systematic review of the literature. *International Journal of Geriatric Psychiatry*, *27*(10), 989–998.

Lejuez, C. W., Hopko, D. R., LePage, J., Hopko, S. D., & McNeil, D. W. (2001). A brief behavioral activation treatment for depression. *Cognitive and Behavioral Practice*, *8*, 164–175.

Lejuez, C. W., Hopko, D. R., Acierno, R., Daughters, S. B, & Pagoto, S. L. (2011). Ten year revision of the brief behavioural activation treatment for depression (BAT-D): revised treatment manual (BATD-R). *Behavior Modification*, *35*, 111–161.

Lenze, E., Mulsant, B., Mohlman, J., Shear, K., Dew, M., Schulz, R., Miller, M., Tracey, B., & Reynolds, C. (2005). Generalized anxiety disorder in late life: lifetime course and comorbidity with major depressive disorder. *The American Journal of Geriatric Psychiatry*, *13*, 77–80.

Levy, B. R. (2003). Mind matters: cognitive and physical effects of aging self-stereotypes. *Journals of Gerontology Series B: Psychological Sciences and Social Sciences*, *58*, 203–211.

Levy, B. R. (2008). Rigidity as a predictor of older persons' aging stereotypes and aging self-perceptions. *Social Behavior and Personality*, *36*, 559–570.

Levy, B. R. (2009). Stereotype embodiment: a psychosocial approach to aging. *Current Directions in Psychological Science*, *18*, 332–336.

Levy, B. R. & Leifheit-Limson, E. (2009). The stereotype-matching effect: Greater influence on functioning when age stereotypes correspond to outcomes. *Psychology & Aging*, *24*, 230–233.

Lewinsohn, P. M., Munoz, R. F., Youngren, M. A., & Zeiss, A. M. (1986). *Control your depression*. New York: Prentice Hall.

Losada, A., Márquez-González, M., Peñacoba, C., & Romero-Moreno, R. (2010). Development and validation of the Caregiver Guilt Questionnaire. *International Psychogeriatrics*, *22*, 650–660.

Lowe, B., Unutzer, J., Callahan, C. M., Perkins, A. J., & Kroenke, K. (2004). Monitoring depression treatment outcomes with the patient health questionnaire-9. *Medical Care*, *42*, 1194–1201.

Luengo-Fernandez, R., Leal, J., & Gray, A. (2010). *Dementia 2010: The economic burden of dementia and associated research funding in the United Kingdom*. Alzheimer's Research Trust.

Liu, R. T. & Alloy, L. B. (2010). Stress generation in depression: a systematic review of the empirical literature and recommendations for future study. *Clinical Psychology, 30*, 582–593.

Lyness, J. M. (2008). Naturalistic outcomes of minor and subsyndromal depression in older primary care patients. *International Journal of Geriatric Psychiatry, 23*, 773–781.

Manthorpe, J. & Moriarty, J. (2010). *Nothing ventured, nothing gained: risk guidance on dementia.* London: Department of Health.

Martell, C. R., Dimidjian, S., & Herman-Dunn, R. (2010). *Behavioral activation for depression: a clinician's guide.* New York: Guilford Press.

McAdams, D. P. (2001). The psychology of life stories. *Review of General Psychology, 5*, 100–122.

McAdams, D. P. (2006) The redemptive self: Generativity and stories Americans live by. *Research in Human Development, 3*, 81-90.

McAdams, D. P. & Adler, J. M. (2010). Autobiographical memory and the construction of a narrative identity. In J. E. Maddux & J. P. Tangney (Eds.), *Social psychological foundations of clinical psychology.* New York: Guilford Press.

McCullough, J. P. (2012). The way early-onset chronically depressed patients are treated today makes me sad. *Open Journal of Psychiatry, 2*, 9–11.

McDougall, F. A., Kvaal, K., Matthews, F. E., Paykel, E., Jones, P. B., Dewey, M. E., & Brayne, C. (2007). Prevalence of depression in older people in England and Wales: The MRC CFA study. *Psychological Medicine, 37*, 1787–1795.

Meyer, T. J., Miller, M. L., Metzger, R. L., & Borkovec, T. D. (1990). Development and validation of the Penn State Worry Questionnaire. *Behaviour Research and Therapy, 28*, 487–495.

Mitchell, A. J., Bird, V., Rizzo, M., & Meader, N. (2010). Diagnostic validity and added value of the Geriatric Depression Scale for depression in primary care: A meta-analysis of the GDS30 and GDS15. *Journal of Affective Disorders, 125*, 10–17.

Mogg, K. & Bradley, P. B. (2005). Attentional bias in generalized anxiety disorder versus depressive disorder. *Cognitive Therapy and Research, 29*, 29–45.

Moher, D., Liberati, A., Tetzlaff, J., & Altman, D. G., The PRISMA Group (2009). Preferred reporting items for systematic reviews and meta-analyses: the PRISMA statement. *PLoS Med, 6*(7), e1000097. doi:10.1371/journal.pmed.1000097.

Mohlman, J. & Gorman, J. M. (2005). The role of executive functioning in CBT: A pilot study with anxious older adults. *Behaviour Research & Therapy, 43*, 447–465.

Monin, J. K. & Schulz, R. (2009). Interpersonal effects of suffering in older adult caregiving relationships. *Psychology & Aging, 24*, 681-695.

Montorio, I., Losada, A., Izal, M., & Marquez, M. (2009). Dysfunctional thoughts about caregiving questionnaire: Psychometric properties of a new measure. *International Psychogeriatrics, 21*, 913–921.

Morin, C. R., Landreville, P., Colecchi, C., McDonald, K., Stone, J., & Ling, W. (1999). The Beck Anxiety Inventory: psychometric properties with older adults. *Journal of Clinical Geropsychology, 5*, 19–29.

NAO, National Audit Office (2011). *Services for people with neurological conditions. Report by the comptroller and auditor general, HC 1586, Session 2010–12.* London: Department of Health, NAO.

Neff, K. D. & Vonk, R. (2009). Self-compassion versus global self-esteem: Two different ways of relating to oneself. *Journal of Personality, 77*, 23–50.

Nelson, W. M. & Politano, P. M. (1993). The goal is to say 'goodbye' and have the treatment effects generalize and maintain: a cognitive-behavioral view of termination. *Journal of Cognitive Psychotherapy, 7*(4), 251–264.

NES, NHS Education for Scotland (2011) The Psychology Matrix. Available at www.nes.scot.nhs.uk/media/20137/Psychology%20Matrix%202013.pdf (accessed August 2014).

Neugarten, B. L., Havinghurst, R. J., & Tobin, S. (1961). The measurement of life satisfaction. *Journal of Gerontology, 16,* 134–143.

NICE, National Institute for Health and Clinical Excellence (2012). *Generalised anxiety disorder in adults: evidence update September 2012.* Manchester: NICE. Available at: www.evidence.nhs.uk/evidence-update-22

Nordhus, I-H. & Pallesen, S. A. (2003). Psychological treatment of late life anxiety: an empirical review. *Journal of Consulting and Clinical Psychology, 71,* 643–651.

Norton, S., Cosco, T., Doyle, F., Done, J., & Sacler, A. (2013). The Hospital and Anxiety Depression Scale: a meta-confirmatory factor analysis. *Journal of Psychosomatic Research, 74,* 74–81.

Nuffield Council on Bioethics (2009). *Dementia: ethical issues.* Cambridge: Nuffield Council on Bioethics.

Ochoa, E. & Muran, J. C. (2008). A relational take on termination in cognitive-behavioral therapy. In W. T. O'Donohue & M. Cucciare (Eds.), *Terminating psychotherapy: a clinician's guide* (pp. 183–204). New York: Routledge.

ONS, Office of National Statistics (2011a). *Older People's Day 2011. Statistical Bulletin.* London: ONS.

ONS, Office of National Statistics (2011b). *Estimates of Centenarians in the UK, 2010. Statistical Bulletin.* London: ONS.

ONS, Office of National Statistics (2011c). *Health expectancies at birth and at age 65 in the United Kingdom, 2007–2009. Statistical Bulletin.* London: ONS.

ONS, Office of National Statistics (2012). *2011 census: population estimates for the United Kingdom, 27 March 2011 (17 December 2012). Statistical Bulletin.* London: ONS.

O'Riordan, T. G., Hayes, J. P., O'Neill, D., Shelley, R., Walsh, J. B., & Coakley, D. (1990). The effect of mild to moderate dementia on the geriatric depression scale and on the general health questionnaire. *Age & Ageing, 19,* 57–61.

Orgeta, V., Spector, A. E., & Orrell, M. (2014). Psychological treatments for depression and anxiety in dementia and mild cognitive impairment. *Cochrane Database of Systematic Reviews, 5,* CD009125. DOI: 10.1002/14651858.CD009125.

Otte, C. (2011). Cognitive behavioural therapy in anxiety disorders: Current state of the evidence. *Dialogues in Clinical Neuroscience, 13,* 413–421.

Overholser, J. C. (1995). Cognitive-behavioral treatment of depression, Part III: reducing cognitive biases. *Journal of Contemporary Psychotherapy, 25,* 311–329.

Overholser, J. C. (1998). Cognitive-behavioral treatment of depression, Part X: reducing the risk of relapse. *Journal of Contemporary Psychotherapy, 28,* 381–396.

Pachana, N. A., Byrne, G. J., Siddle, H., Koloski, N., Harley, E., & Arnold, E. (2007). Development and validation of the Geriatric Anxiety Inventory. *International Psychogeriatrics, 19,* 103–114.

Padesky, C. A. (1993). Socratic questioning: changing minds or guided discovery? Paper presented at the European Congress of Behavioural and Cognitive Therapies, London.

Padesky, C. A. & Mooney, K. A. (1990). Presenting the cognitive model to clients. *International Cognitive Therapy Newsletter, 6*, 13–14.

Palmqvist, S., Hannsson, O., Minthon, L., & Londos, E. (2009). Practical suggestions on how to differentiate dementia with Lewy bodies from Alzheimer's disease with common cognitive tests. *International Journal of Geriatric Psychiatry, 24*, 1405–1412.

Paukert, A. L., Calleo, J., Kraus-Schuman, C., Snow, L., Wilson, N., Petersen, N. J., Kunik, M. E., & Stanley, M. A. (2010). Peaceful mind: an open trial of cognitive-behavioral therapy for anxiety in persons with dementia. *International Psychogeriatrics, 22*, 1012–1021.

Persons, J. B. (1989). *Cognitive therapy in practice: A case formulation approach.* New York: W. W. Norton & Co.

Persons, J. B. (2008). *The case formulation approach to cognitive-behavior therapy.* New York: Guilford Press.

Pinquart, M. & Sorensen, S. (2001). How effective are psychotherapeutic and other psychosocial interventions with older adults? A meta-analysis. *Journal of Mental Health and Aging, 7*, 207–243.

Pinquart, M., & Sorensen, S. (2006). Helping caregivers of persons with dementia: which interventions work and how large are their effects? *International Psychogeriatrics, 18*, 577–595.

Pinquart, M. & Sorensen, S. (2011). Spouses, adult children, and children-in-law as caregivers of older adults: a meta-analytic comparison. *Psychology & Aging, 26*, 1–14.

Pinquart, M., Duberstein, P. R., & Lyness, J. M. (2006). Treatments for later-life depressive conditions: a meta-analytic comparison of pharmacotherapy and psychotherapy. *American Journal of Psychiatry, 163*, 1493–1501.

Pinquart, M., Duberstein, P., & Lyness, J. (2007). Effects of psychotherapy and other behavioural interventions on clinically depressed older adults: a meta analysis. *Aging & Mental Health, 11*, 645–657.

Pruchno, R. (2012). Special issue: baby boomers. not your mother's old age: baby boomers at age 65. *The Gerontologist, 52*, 149–152.

Quinn, K. M., Laidlaw, K., Murray, L. K. (2009). Older peoples' attitudes to mental illness. *Clinical Psychology and Psychotherapy, 16*, 33–45.

RCP, Royal College of Psychiatrists (2012). *Individual patient outcome measures recommended for use in older people's mental health.* Prepared by the Royal College of Psychiatrists' Faculty of the Psychiatry of Old Age. Occasional Paper, OP86, October 2012. London: RCP.

Rinaldi, P., Mecocci, P., Bendetti, C., Ercolani, S., Bregnocchi, M., Menculini, G., Catani, M., Senin, U., & Cherubini, A. (2003). Validation of the five-item Geriatric Depression Scale in elderly subjects in three different settings. *Journal of the American Geriatrics Society, 51*, 694–698.

Roach, L., Laidlaw, K., Gillanders, D., & Quinn, K. (2013). Validation of the Caregiver Guilt Questionnaire (CGQ) in a sample of British dementia caregivers. *International Psychogeriatrics, 25*(12), 2001–2010.

Robinson, L., Gemski, A., Abley, A., Bond, J., Keady, J., Campbell, S., Samsi, K., & Manthorpe, J. (2011). The transition to dementia – individual and family experiences of receiving a diagnosis: a review. *International Psychogeriatrics, 23*, 1026–1034.

Richardson, T. & Marshall, A. (2012). Cognitive behavioural therapy for depression in advanced Parkinson's disease: a case illustration. *The Cognitive Behaviour Therapist, 5*, 60–69.

Roth, A. D. & Pilling, S. (2007). *The competences required to deliver effective cognitive and behavioural therapy for people with depression and anxiety disorders.* London: Department of Health.

Rozario, P. A., Kidahashi, M., & DeRienzis, D. R. (2011). Selection, optimization and compensation: strategies to maintain, maximize and generate resources in late life in the face of chronic illnesses. *Journal of Gerontological Social Work, 54*, 224–239.

Rybarczyk, B., Gallagher-Thompson, D., Rodman, J., Zeiss, A., Gantz, F. E., & Yesavage, J. (1992). Applying cognitive-behavioral psychotherapy to the chronically ill elderly: treatment issues and case illustration. *International Psychogeriatrics, 4*, 127–140.

Sadavoy, J. (2009). An integrated model for defining the scope of psychogeriatrics: The five Cs. *International Psychogeriatrics, 21*, 805–812.

Safran, J. & Segal, Z. (1996). *Interpersonal process in cognitive therapy.* New Jersey: Jason Aronson.

Salkovskis, P., Clark, D. M., Hackmann, A., Wells, A., & Gelder, M. G. (1999). An experimental investigation of the role of safety-seeking behaviours in the maintenance of panic disorder with agoraphobia. *Behaviour, Research & Therapy, 37*, 559–574.

Samad, Z., Brealey, S., & Gilbody, S. (2011). The effectiveness of behavioural therapy for the treatment of depression in older adults: a meta-analysis. *International Journal of Geriatric Psychiatry, 26*, 1211–1220.

Scheibe, S. & Carstensen, L. (2010). Emotional aging: recent findings and future trends. *Journals of Gerontology Series B: Psychological Sciences and Social Sciences, 65*, 135–144.

Scholey, K. A. & Woods, B. T. (2003). A series of brief cognitive therapy interventions with people experiencing both dementia and depression. *Clinical Psychology and Psychotherapy, 10*, 175–185.

Scogin, F. & Shah, A. (Eds.). (2012). *Making evidence-based psychological treatments work with older adults.* Washington, DC: APA.

Scogin, F., Welsh, D., Hanson, A., Stump, J., & Coates, A. (2005). Evidence-based psychotherapies for depression in older adults. *Clinical Psycholology: Science and Practice, 12*, 222–237.

Scott, T., MacKenzie, C. S., Chipperfield, J. G., & Sareen, J. (2010). Mental health service use among Canadian older adults with anxiety disorders and clinically significant anxiety symptoms. *Aging & Mental Health, 14*, 790–800.

Segal, D. L., Coolidge, F. L., Cahil, B. S., & O'Riley, A. A. (2008). Psychometric properties of the Beck Depression Inventory-II (BDI-II) among community-dwelling older adults. *Behavior Modification, 32*, 3–20.

Segal, D. L., June, A., Payne, M., Coolidge, F. L., & Yochim, B. (2010). Development and initial validation of a self-report assessment tool for anxiety among older adults: the geriatric anxiety scale. *Journal of Anxiety Disorders, 24*, 709–714.

Selwood, A., Johnston, K., Katona, C., Lyketsos, C., & Livingston, G. (2007). Systematic review of the effect of psychological interventions for family caregivers of people with dementia. *Journal of Affective Disorders, 101*, 75–89.

Serfaty, M., Haworth, D., Blanchard, M., Buszewicz, M., Murad, S., & King, M. (2009). Clinical effectiveness of individual cognitive behavioural therapy for depressed older people in primary care. *Archives of General Psychiatry, 66*, 1332–1340.

Serfaty, M., Csipke, E., Haworth, D., Murad, S., & King, M. (2011). A talking control for use in evaluating the effectiveness of cognitive-behavioral therapy. *Behaviour Research & Therapy, 49,* 433–440.

Shah, A., Lewis, H. S., Mahendran, S. L., Platt, J., & Battacharyya, B. (1997). Screening for depression among acutely ill geriatric inpatients with a short geriatric depression scale. *Age and Ageing, 26,* 217–221.

Shenkin, S., Laidlaw, K., Allerhand, M., Mead, G. E., Starr, J. M., & Deary, I. (2014). Life course influences of physical and cognitive function on Attitudes to Ageing in the Lothian Birth Cohort 1936. *International Psychogeriatrics, 26*(9), 1417–1430.

Sivrioglu, E. Y., Sivrioglu, K., Ertan, T., Ertan, S. F., Cankurtaran, E., Aki, O., Uluduz, D., Ince, B., & Kirli, S. (2009). Reliability and validity of the geriatric depression scale in detection of poststroke minor depression. *Journal of Clinical & Experimental Neuropsychology, 31,* 999–1006.

Sorocco, K. H. & Lauderdale, S. (2011). *Cognitive behavior therapy with older adults: innovation across care settings.* New York: Springer.

Spector, A., Orrell, M., Charlesworth, G., Qazi, S., Hoe, J., Hardwood, K., & King, M. (2013). *I can't forget to worry: a pilot randomized controlled trial of CBT for anxiety in people with dementia.* NIHR, Research for Patient Benefit (FrPB). Programme, Final Report Form.

Spitzer, R. L., Kroenke, K., & Williams, J. B. W., for the Patient Health Questionnaire Primary Care Study Group (1999). Validation and utility of a self-report version of PRIME-MD: the PHQ Primary Care Study. *Journal of the American Medical Association, 282,* 1737–1744.

Spitzer, R. L., Kroenke, K., Williams, J. B. W., & Löwe, B. (2006). A brief measure for assessing generalized anxiety disorder: the GAD-7. *Archives of Internal Medicine, 166,* 1092–1097.

Stanley, M. A., Novy, D. M., Bourland, S. L., Beck, J. G., & Averill, P. M. (2001). Assessing older adults with generalized anxiety: a replication and extension. *Behaviour Research & Therapy, 39,* 221–235.

Stanley, M. A., Wilson, N. L., & Novy, D. M., et al. (2009). Cognitive behavior therapy for generalized anxiety disorder among older adults in primary care: a randomized controlled trial. *Journal of the American Medical Association, 301,* 1460–1467.

Staudinger, U. & Glück, J. (2011). Psychological wisdom research: commonalities and differences in a growing field. *Annual Review of Psychology, 62,* 215–241.

Sternberg, R. J. (2012). The science of wisdom: implications for psychotherapy. In C. K. Germer & R. D. Siegel (Eds.), *Wisdom and compassion in psychotherapy: Deepening mindfulness in clinical practice.* New York: Guilford Press Inc.

Teri, L. (1994). Behavioral treatment of depression in patients with dementia. *Alzheimer's Disease and Associated Disorders, 8,* (Suppl. 3), 66–74.

Teri, L., Logsdon, R. G., Uomoto, J., McCurry, S. M. (1997). Behavioral treatment of depression in dementia patients: a controlled clinical trial. *The Journals of Gerontology Series B: Psychological Sciences and Social Sciences, 52,* 159–166.

Thorp, S. R., Ayers, C. R., Nuevo, R., Stoddard, J. A., Sorrell, J. T., & Wetherell, J. L. (2009). Meta-analysis comparing different behavioural treatments for late life anxiety. *The American Journal of Geriatric Psychiatry, 17,* 105–115.

Tompkins, M. A. (2002). Guidelines for enhancing homework compliance. *JCLP/In session: Psychotherapy in Practice, 58*, 565–576.

Troeung, L., Egan, S. J., & Gasson, N. (2013). A meta-analysis of randomized placebo-controlled treatment trials for depression and anxiety in Parkinson's disease. *PLoS One, 8*(11), e79510.

UN, Department of Economic and Social Affairs, Population Division (2011). *World population prospects: the 2010 revision, Highlights and advance tables.* Working Paper No. ESA/P/WP.220.

UNFPA, United Nations Population Fund and HelpAge International (2012). *Ageing in the twenty-first century: a celebration and a challenge.* New York: UNFPA.

Unutzer, J., Katon, W., Sullivan, M., & Miranda J. (1999). Treating depressed older adults in primary care: narrowing the gap between efficacy and effectiveness. *Milbank Quarterly, 77*, 225–256.

Vernooij-Dassen, M., Drasovic, I., McCleery, J., & Downs, M. (2011). Cognitive reframing for carers of people with dementia. *The Cochrane Database of Systematic Reviews*, CD005318.

Vink, D., Aartsen, M. J., & Schoevers, R. A. (2008). Risk factors for anxiety and depression in the elderly: a review. *Journal of Affective Disorders, 106*, 27–44.

Walker, D. A. (2004). Cognitive behavioural therapy for depression in a person with Alzheimer's dementia. *Behavioural & Cognitive Psychotherapy, 32*, 495–500.

Waller, G. (2009). Evidence-based treatment and therapist drift. *Behaviour Research & Therapy, 47*, 119–127.

Wampold, B. E., Budge, S. L., Laska, K. M., Del Re, A. C., Baardseth, T. P., Fluckiger, C., Minami, T., Kivlighan, D. M., & Gunn, W. (2011). Evidence-based treatments for depression and anxiety versus treatment as usual: a meta-analysis of direct comparisons. *Clinical Psychology Review, 31*, 1304–1312.

Wancata, J., Alexandrowicz, R., Marquet, B., Weiss, M., Freidrich, F. (2006). The criterion validity of the Geriatric Depression Scale: a systematic review. *Acta Psychiatrica Scandinavica, 114*, 398–410.

Watkins, E. R., Baeyens, C. B., & Read, R. (2009). Concreteness training reduces dysphoria: proof-of-principle for repeated cognitive bias modification in depression. *Journal of Abnormal Psychology, 118*, 55–64.

Wetherell, J. L. & Gatz, M. (2005). The Beck Anxiety Inventory in Older Adults with generalized anxiety disorder. *Journal of Psychopathology and Behavioral Assessment, 27*, 17–24.

Wetherell, J. L., Lenze, E., & Stanley, M. A. (2005). Evidence-based treatment of geriatric anxiety disorders. *Psychiatric Clinics of North America, 28*, 871–896.

WHO (1980). *International classification of impairments, disabilities and handicaps.* Geneva: WHO.

WHO (2012). *Dementia: A public health priority.* Geneva: WHO.

Wild, B., Eckl, A., Herzog, W., Niehoff, D., Lechner, S., Maatouk, I., Schellberg, D., Brenner, H., Muller, H., & Lowe, B. (2013). Assessing Generalized Anxiety Disorder in elderly people using the GAD-7 and GAD-2 scales: Results of a validation study. *American Journal of Geriatric Psychiatry.* doi: 10.1016/j.jagp.2013.01.076.

Wilkins, P. (2000). Unconditional positive regard reconsidered. *British Journal of Guidance and Counselling, 28*, 23–36.

Williams, L. S., Brizendine, M. S., Plue, L., Bakas, T., Tu, W., Hendrie, H., & Kroenke, K. (2005). Performance of the PHQ-9 as a screening tool for depression after stroke. *Stroke, 36*, 635–638.

Wilson, K., Mottram, P., & Vassilas, C. (2008). Psychotherapeutic treatments for older depressed people. *Cochrane Database of Systematic Reviews, 1.* Art. No.: CD004853. doi: 10.1002/14651858.CD0044853.pub2.

Wolitzky-Taylor, K. B., Castriotta, N., Lenze, E. J., Stanley, M. A., & Craske, M. G. (2010). Anxiety disorders in older adults: a comprehensive review. *Depression and Anxiety, 27*, 190–211.

Worden, J. W. (2009). *Grief counseling and grief therapy* (4th ed.). New York: Springer.

Yesavage, J. A., Brink, T. L., Rose, T. L., Lum, O., Huang, V., Adey, M. B., & Leirer, V. O. (1983). Development and validation of a geriatric depression screening scale. *Journal of Psychiatric Research, 39*, 37–49.

Yochim, B., Mueller, A. E., June, A., & Segal, D. L. (2011). Psychometric properties of the Geriatric Anxiety Scale: comparison to the Beck Anxiety Inventory and Geriatric Anxiety Inventory. *Clinical Gerontologist, 34*, 21–33.

Zeiss, A. & Steffen, A. (1996). Treatment issues with elderly clients. *Cognitive and Behavioral Practice, 3*, 371–389.

Zigmond, A. S. & Snaith, R. P. (1983). The hospital anxiety and depression scale. *Acta Psychiatrica Scandinavica, 67*, 361–370.

Index